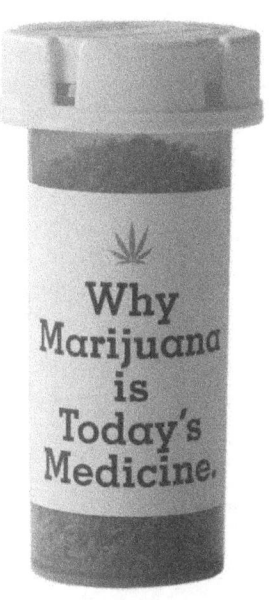

Why
Marijuana
is
Today's
Medicine.

Pot Luck.

Why
Marijuana
is
Today's
Medicine.

RICHARD W. LEWIS

MIKHAIL J. ARTAMONOV, MD

DahlenDesign

Also by Richard W. Lewis

WHY HIRE JENNIFER?

How to Use Branding and Uncommon Sense
to Get Your First Job, Last Job,
and every Job in Between.

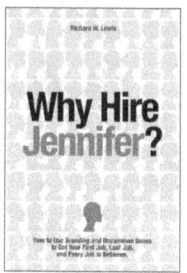

ABSOLUT BOOK.

The Absolut Vodka Advertising Story.

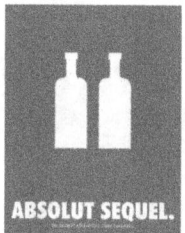

ABSOLUT SEQUEL.

The Absolut Advertising Story Continues.

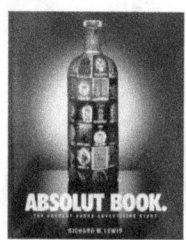

Also by Mikhail J. Artamonov

YOUR HEALTH, YOUR WEIGHT, YOUR LIFE.
A Good Medicine | Weight Loss Guide.

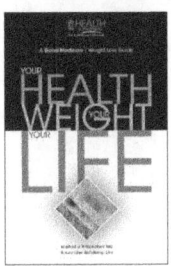

HEALTH IS EVERYTHING.
Patients, Practitioners and Good Medicine.

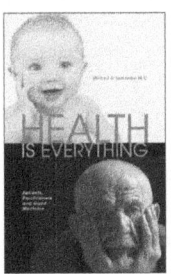

Dedicated to the Patients,
who are just looking for a normal day.

Pot Luck.

Why Marijuana is The Next Impactful Medicine

Richard W. Lewis & Mikhail J. Artamonov, MD

RL Ideas, Ltd.
256 Clinton Avenue
Dobbs Ferry, NY 10522

Printed by CreateSpace, An Amazon.com Company

More information at potluckbook.me

To report errors, please send a note to rl@rlconsulting.biz

Copyright © 2015 by Richard W. Lewis & Mikhail J. Artamonov, MD

Book Designer: Juergen Dahlen

ISBN. 978-1511447706

Printed and bound in the United States of America.

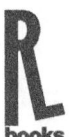
books

Contents

Tracy Monte
Upstate, NY

Tracy Monte just might be the frankest person I've ever met.

She grew up in East New York – that's Brooklyn. Before quitting high school her passion was playing softball, third base, the hot corner. She earned her G.E.D. in 1979 and attended Queensboro Community College. Upon graduation she took all the civil service exams: sanitation, police, bridge and tunnels.

"Since I was gay I knew I needed to take care of myself and that meant a dependable job."

Tracy was a pot smoker as a teenager but gave it up when she joined the force. After serving as a NY Transit officer she joined the NYPD, working on the Lower East Side in the Neighborhood Stabilization Unit during "Operation Pressure Point." As this was the 1980s, it wasn't a pretty job, as the LES wasn't the up and coming neighborhood it is today. It was more like down and going, with drugs, crime, and other unpleasantness.

Later, working in Queens during days, she then served a second shift in Crown Heights during the demonstrations and riots, as it was all hands on deck.

"You have to have a certain amount of fear as a police officer, otherwise you get killed."

Tracy was injured on the job a couple of times in scuffles with suspects before she was attacked in a stairway, one morning in 1992 by a drunk building super, tumbling the rest of the way down, all because she was intervening in a landlord-tenant dispute.

For her effort she earned a titanium plate in her neck, as well as two broken shoulders. Placed on sick leave, then on modified duty, Tracy retired on disability the following year.

But the pain and anxiety didn't retire even as she returned to work, first in security at Adelphi University and then as a massage therapist. On the plus side, she married her partner, Robin, in Canada in 2006.

During couples' therapy a few years later the therapist

asked if she had ever been diagnosed with PTSD. Tracy's symptoms, fear of crowds, bad dreams, and obsession with her personal space, were aligned with that diagnosis. The bell rang in her mind: "That's why I'm like this."

Tracy's now daily regimen of cannabis – cookies, muffins, and peanut butter – are her kitchen medicine cabinet. And besides the occasional Naproxen, for the "big pain," she's doing quite well.

Their house is up for sale as they are set to become Colorado refugees. She wants to increase her activist role in Law Enforcement Against Prohibition (LEAP) in a more sympathetic environment. She says this is a growing movement, police officers unhappy policing people's drug habits. Plus she adds, proudly, "I never busted anyone for weed."

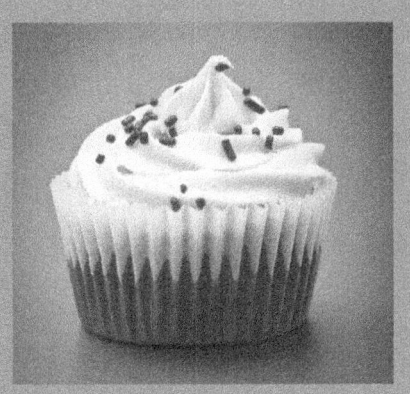

Introduction.

When I was first introduced to marijuana in the late 1960s I don't recall any medical conversation. Yes, there was a bell curve of energy, excitement, headiness, and appetite that ultimately produced a peaceful, laid-back sleepiness, and then, ultimately, sleep.

Ah, sleep, merciful sleep. What so many people would give for a simple good night's sleep, just a night without pain, nausea, anxiety, and uncontrolled thoughts. Sleep, then the side effect, is now the central effect desired by millions.

I didn't know anything about marijuana back then, fortunately, some other people did. Marijuana has been growing for thousands of years and had been used as a medicine just as long, before the near-hysterical Reefer Madness chorus in America culminated in its designation as a Schedule I drug in 1970. (More on that significance later.)

It's time to be positive. As of this writing, and it

changes very fast, 23 states have legalized medical marijuana, and like an electronic scoreboard, that number needs to be updated frequently. Four states – Colorado, Oregon, Alaska and Washington – have gone one big step further and legalized recreational marijuana for every adult. This is incredible progress.

Because back in the 1970s, many people, including me, thought that marijuana would be legalized within five years. Of course, that didn't happen, but I still felt it would happen, so I looked at it as a rolling five-year prediction. Every year it was still just five years away, very imaginable.

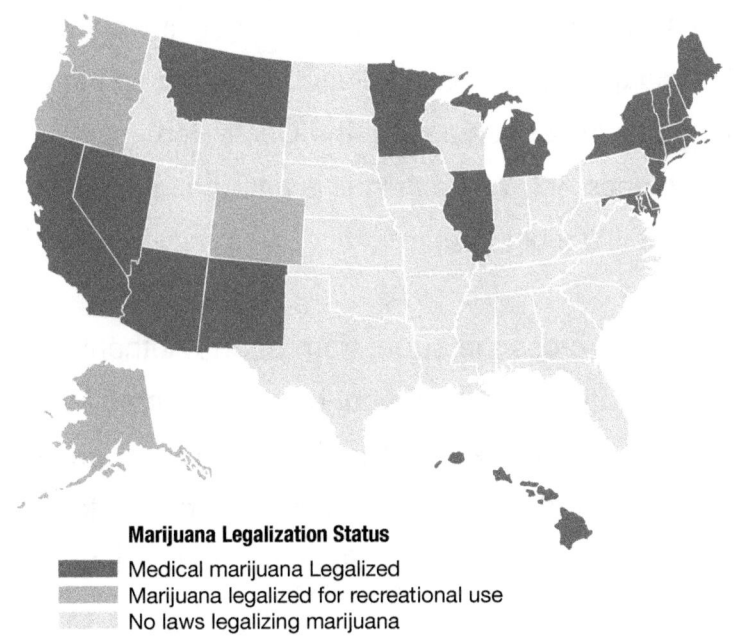

Marijuana Legalization Status

Medical marijuana Legalized
Marijuana legalized for recreational use
No laws legalizing marijuana

Clearly, that day is now. The distribution of legal medical marijuana states and likely medical marijuana states looks like a pending Election Night victory. And, yes, it's still a hodgepodge of laws, and federally the drug is still illegal – not unlike same sex marriage – but that's why the founding fathers protected states' rights, too. My point is, all arrows are pointing up, and people who need or want medical marijuana soon won't have to run a Survivor course to obtain it.

Consider: Three U.S. Senators – two Democrats and one Republican – introduced a bill in March 2015 that would eliminate the threat of federal prosecution in states where medical marijuana is legal. It would also shift marijuana from the radioactive Schedule I to the half glass full Schedule II of the Controlled Substances Act. While the bill is a tough journey to passage it's a big deal.

Consider: Across the street from Sports Authority Stadium in Denver, Colorado, better known as Mile High Stadium, is the Mile High Marijuana Dispensary. And while Stadium owners declare it verboten to use marijuana in or around the Stadium – hey, it is their property – you can imagine there are more than a few scofflaws.

Consider: State Senators Daylin Leach and Mike Folmer, representing Pennsylvania's 17th and 4th districts, respectively, a bi-partisan team, no less, are reintroducing SB 1182 and are optimistic that Tom Wolf, recently elected governor will sign it. Leach believes, "Anyone can get sick, anyone can have a relative get sick, and legislators shouldn't be making lists of conditions and medicines tying up doctors' hands."

Consider: Last summer I was in Laguna Beach, California, a medical marijuana state since 1996, when I came across a couple vaping; that is, ingesting marijuana through a vaporizer outside the local candy (real candy, as in Tootsie Rolls) store. I wouldn't even have noticed if my daughter, who has a nose for this stuff, hadn't pointed them out. Speaking of vaping, "vape" was the 2014 Oxford Dictionary "Word of the Year."

Which leads to the not-so-profound thought that there is a handshake occurring between recreational marijuana and medical marijuana. As medical marijuana states evolve into legal states the mixing of stoners and patients will likely obscure, perhaps erase, each label, and I think that is for the better.

However, what still passes for conventional wisdom among the uninformed is the belief that medical marijuana cannot be medical if it's also fun. And it can't be medical if it's against the law. And it can't be safe if so many people say it isn't. But try to find a single death attributable to a marijuana overdose. Serious people have tried but can't. (While six Americans die daily from alcohol poisoning according to the Centers for Disease Control.)

It's difficult, if not impossible, to discuss medical marijuana without recreational marijuana barging in. Think of it as the green elephant in the room. Because serious-minded, health-oriented people, particularly patients, doctors, and their loved ones, have to contend with the political, business, legal, medical, and eyebrow-raising moralizers, too, as they go about their quest for relief, to experience a normal day.

When you speak to the patients it's not an exaggeration to describe their quixotic quests for help.

I reached out to medical marijuana patients around the country to learn how they became patients; to learn what maladies or illnesses they suffered from, what doctors and treatments they used before, until they finally – in many cases – spun the medical game spinner and asked, "Why not marijuana?"
I also spoke to doctors to discover what led them to recommend such an unorthodox and politically charged treatment, often risking their professional licenses and reputations.

Nearly all these individuals, doctors and patients, have gone on record, using their actual names and locales. Where they needed to be anonymous, for whatever personal or professional reasons, I have made that clear, too.

Heidi Whitman
San Diego, CA

Heidi Whitman is 25 years old and lives in San Diego. In 2006, as a 17-year old student, she was a passenger on a pleasure boat in Boston when it hit a huge rogue wave, went airborne, and then crashed back into the water.

Heidi, too, went flying into the air, landing back on the deck, smack on her face. She suffered a compound fracture of her jaw and broke several teeth.

Over the course of many restorative surgeries and the continuous use of painkillers, Heidi developed severe anxiety, which led to cyclic vomiting syndrome.

"It's even worse than it sounds. Cyclic vomiting releases everything you eat, drink, until all you can do is retch, retch, retch," she told me.

She had no appetite, retained very little food when able to eat, and lost a great deal of weight. She describes it as a constantly knotty stomach. Unable to focus, she had to drop out of college. Heidi's gastroenterologist recommended she try medical marijuana. But as it wasn't yet available in Massachusetts, she moved to California. The results were immediate: no more vomiting, a healthy appetite, and she soon regained the lost weight. She smokes, vapes, and eats edibles. Her marijuana of choice is a hybrid offering both sedation and uplift, preferring strains such as Bubba Kush, and Afghani.

Today Heidi works for a non-profit medical marijuana business and says, "It's good to be normal and accepted; it's good to be me."

Chapter

1

Why Another Marijuana Book?

It's late summer, 2014. I'm getting ready to return to NYU where I teach an Honors Seminar to incoming Freshmen – students who I refer to as having left high school just fifteen minutes ago. I'm a one-person department in the College of Arts and Sciences where I teach a course on Branding, which you may know is a slice of marketing devoted to how consumers think about businesses, countries, politicians and themselves. Which makes sense because I am a self-described "Marketing Guy," a title I admit encompasses a number of garden-variety sins but also enables me to operate under the radar to ask and answer some of the bigger questions about careers, medicine, religion, and culture. I had recently published a new book, "Why Hire Jennifer?" a branding and job search guide for college students and their nervous parents. (Having been a nervous parent, I possess all the pre-requisites.)

Mikhail Artamonov, the poly-doc.

I received an out-of-the-blue e-mail from a client and friend, Dr. Mikhail Artamonov, whom I've known for about five years. Mikhail is a physiatrist. Not a

psychiatrist, but a physiatrist, which is a physician –
M.D. – who specializes in physical medicine and
rehabilitation. One of the many things that make him
special, he's a poly-doc, someone who has an
appetite for everything in the pursuit of good
medicine.

Mikhail received a medical degree in Moscow – where
he is from – but also pursued advanced training both
in the U.S. and later, in China. He's board certified in
pain management, physical medicine and he is board
eligible (completed all requirements) in addiction
medicine, electrodiagnostic medicine, medical
acupuncture, and functional and anti-aging medicine.
Hence, the poly.

He practices integrated medicine, employing methods
from his wide and extensive training. This contributes
to making him a very open-minded doctor, not
wedded to a particular orthodoxy or rulebook. He's
interested in results and happy patients, which usually
travel together.

The e-mail suggested: "Let's do a medical marijuana book. Interested?"

Dr. Artamonov practices in Pennsylvania and New York, states still on the cusp of implementing medical marijuana. But he was looking around the corner.

My initial thoughts were, I don't know anything about medical marijuana, except its ability to relieve the nausea brought about by chemotherapy. (And that I learned just from watching TV.) Then I thought about what I'm skilled at and enjoy: research, analysis, brainstorming, and creative implementation. That's my marketing training. Plus, I'm a bit of a fireman on the lookout for the next fire.

"Yes, I don't know anything, but I'm interested."

But do we really need another medical marijuana book?

That's the question I asked myself. Because if I were to tackle this project, I would have to believe I could at the very least add something to the conversation and that time spent on it would be meaningful. I can still recall from my ad agency days the marketing plan tomes that clients spent hundreds of man-hours assembling with great care and effort only to be then placed on their office shelves like large ceramic bears, to be admired but never even cracked open.

A quick check of Amazon reveals hundreds of books on marijuana. I bought a few, even read them, and concluded, like any controversial subject in the spotlight, there are books written by experts and books written by people posing as experts. There is useful information and there is useless information. There are people who want to cash in and people who genuinely want to help. (I have included a few recommendations at the end of the book.)

At about the same time I had an appointment with my ophthalmologist. I asked if he was familiar with the benefits of medical marijuana for treating glaucoma. He eagerly told a story about a patient of his who takes glaucoma eye drops and smokes marijuana.

"His eye pressures are great taking both. I just don't know how it would be if he stopped taking the drops."

I asked if he was curious what would happen if the patient stopped taking the drops.

"Of course I'm curious, but I'm a doctor. If this regimen works I'm not going to alter it. Not to mention, medical marijuana isn't legal yet in New York. Or is it?"

That last sentence summarizes much of today's state of medical marijuana practice: If conventional medicine – drugs, surgery, and therapy – work, stick with the program. If medical marijuana is added to the treatment and doesn't "hurt," then, why not?

If it's an issue of legality, it casts a cloud over the entire conversation and the decision.

We continued talking for a few minutes until it was time for him to see another patient. Standing up, he said, "Sounds like you know more than I do."

Walking out I thought, "Well, that's kind of crazy. I don't know anything."

Perhaps, I know more than I thought. Because we have a tendency, particularly for serious stuff like our health, our family, our money, to be drawn toward the rules and guidelines we acquired growing up. In particular, the lessons we learned when we were young and most impressionable. (Most eight year olds aren't yet cynical.)

Our fathers take us to baseball games long before we understand the benefit of the sacrifice bunt. Our parents try to teach us the "value" of money and values of money: Don't buy all the crap you see in the stores. Doctors and auto mechanics know how to fix anything if we just give them the opportunity. We seek their expertise.

But a larger issue is at play: If I had been raised in, say, Long Ben Phu, in China, instead of Long Island, New York, Eastern medicine would have been my native treatment, not an alternative when everything else, everything Western, failed. We aren't accustomed to thinking of using marijuana as a treatment when an illness is first identified. We are accustomed to trying unconventional treatments when all else has failed.

Or we live with disturbing or dangerous side effects if the conventional treatment works up to the point the side effects are worse than the disease.

I'm in awe that middle class "Easterners" – Chinese, Korean, Japanese, for instance – continue to use traditional Eastern methods for treating illness and maintaining well being that doesn't begin with prescription medicine and conclude with surgery.

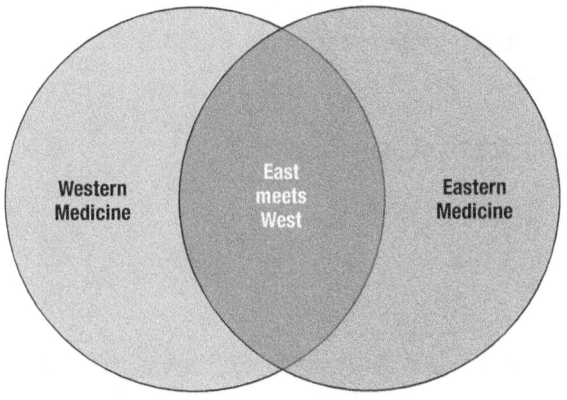

In the United States practitioners of Traditional Chinese Medicine (TCM) have to conform to the same laws as the medical establishment, which means it varies state to state. TCM does not classify

THC, the component in marijuana that makes us high, as part of their materia medica. However, they use marijuana seeds because there's no THC in the seeds, because it's applicable for many different ailments and is extremely safe for even pregnant or nursing mothers. Acupuncturists use it in states where it is legal and most I spoke to plan to use it when it becomes legal.

Yet, medical marijuana is also a pariah in much of the Asian medical establishment more because of its criminal association, than because doctors don't believe in its effectiveness.

Will this book be relevant in 2025?

Frankly, I doubt it.

Because that will mean society's laws will have caught up with society. It will mean medical marijuana will be legal everywhere. It will mean doctors are using it as part of their patient regimen without fear of risking their reputations and livelihood. It will mean patients will have easy access to both the supply of medical marijuana and the expertise on when and how to use it.

Then, too, the lines between recreation and therapy will become more blurred, as medical marijuana will be considered as a healthy life enhancer, maybe right on the order of magnitude of diet, exercise, and sleep, superior to red wine, and likely above many addicting and toxic prescription drugs.

As it's still illegal in half the country, most patients have neither the access to the medical marijuana nor the medical expertise to dispense it. Sure, patients can move from Texas to Colorado, for instance, but unless the suffering is approaching the unbearable, this isn't a ready solution for most people.

Whether or not 2025 looks like 2015 on the medical marijuana landscape, the stories of the patients and practitioners on the front lines, whose lives have dramatically changed for the better when they discovered medical marijuana, will remain relevant.

Dr. Lester Grinspoon
Wellesley, MA

It's a severe understatement to describe Lester
Grinspoon, MD as the "father of marijuana."
He's actually the father, grandfather, mother, uncle,
cousin and next-door neighbor.

Even back in college in the 1970s I was familiar with
his name. He rose to national attention with his
publication of *Marijuana Reconsidered* in 1971. Why
reconsidered? Because Grinspoon set out to squash
pot's growing popularity, particularly among youth, by
demonstrating its harmful effects, only to discover
virtually no empirical evidence about its dangers.

Grinspoon's credentials – Harvard Medical School,
Massachusetts Medical Health Center (Boston) as
Senior Psychiatrist, American Association of the
Advancement of Science Fellow – lent a gravitas to a
wing of medicine that up to then had been, well,
weightless.

Medical marijuana has been his life's work.

He surely could have chosen something less controversial as he is a brilliant scientist and doctor who, at 86 years old, is still fighting the good fight. He writes, he advocates, and he talks, from his basement office in Wellesley.

And he bemoans the state of modern marijuana medicine.

"Today, only 7% of doctors would agree to write a prescription for cannabinopathic medicine. What's the story with the other 93%? It's a safe drug, effective drug. It's just shameful," he told me.

But because there's no money in it for Big Pharma, increased use of medical marijuana actually works against the drug business, substituting for opium-derived products.

Yet Grinspoon isn't a one-eyed evangelist. He preaches the combination of medical marijuana and chemotherapy not just because it curbs the nausea, enabling patients to eat more, but because he says the marijuana helps suppress tumor metastasis. (While he's

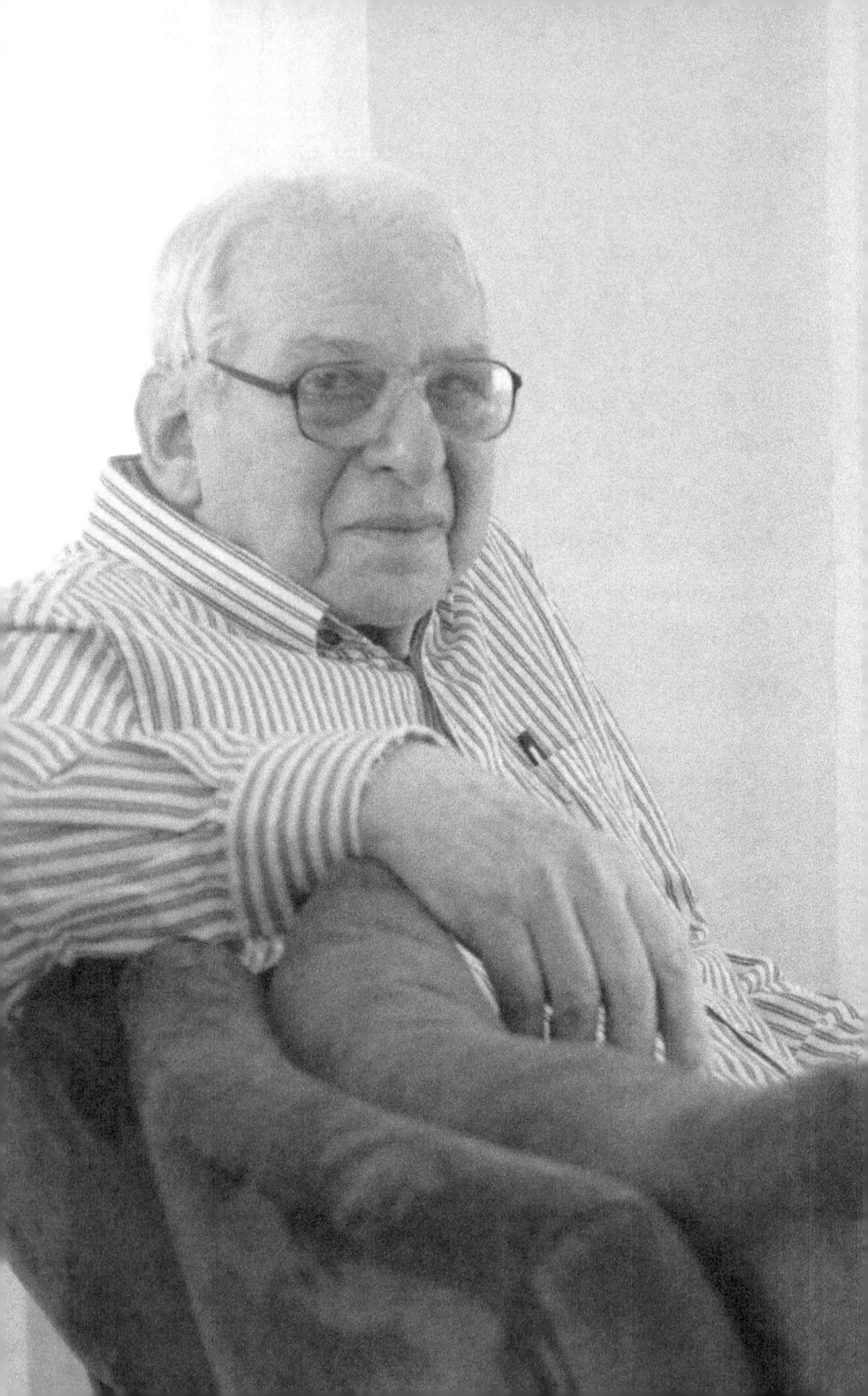

not alone in this belief, it's still an aggressive one.)

This he learned firsthand as a cancer survivor. And he learned that medical marijuana relieved some of the ordeal his teenage son, Danny, endured before succumbing to cancer.

Right now he has to go. His wife Betsy wants him to stop working and join her for a walk. I encourage him to go. There'll be another chance to talk about his favorite subject.

2

What's So Bad About Feeling Good?

If you're someone who has never tried marijuana you may have been overwhelmed by all the noise, and there is certainly plenty.

Legal.

Certainly a consideration, even as marijuana use, possession, and distribution is decriminalized in more and more states.

Social.

Fear of not being in full control of yourself, fear of feeling uncomfortable, fear that it just may not work for you.

Indifference.

Perhaps, you simply have little interest in trying it, just as you may have little interest in eating sushi.

Ignorance.

Perhaps, you didn't know until now – or still may have reservations about using medical marijuana for your malady.

Marijuana and medical marijuana don't "work' for

everyone. Often ingesting marijuana requires a few trials for your body to become accustomed to it and for you to determine a proper dosage. Which really isn't much different when a doctor prescribes a new medication that requires a few weeks to determine its effectiveness.

Yes, we are a hurry-up, speed-up, get-out-of-my-way nation, where the car behind us hits the horn as the light turns green, but the body adheres to its own timetable and is a little mellower than the guy in the Jeep.

The speed of the reaction is also determined by how you ingest:

■ Combustion (smoking),

■ Vaporization,

■ Sublingual (under the tongue) or swallowing.

■ Topical application

And it's also determined by the type of medical marijuana you purchase. While choosing a strain isn't yet as exacting as choosing a wine, there is already a snob appeal among the cognoscenti, because the variety of strains and brands is pretty remarkable. We will discuss this in the following chapters.

But in the meantime, feel free to close your eyes and imagine yourself feeling good, having a sense of well-being, and heightened sensory antenna: seeing, smelling, tasting.

And feeling better about your illness, pain, sleeplessness, and anxiety, by reducing their symptoms and even providing a measure of healing.

Teri Robnett

Denver, CO

Teri Robnett is the Founder and Executive Director of the Cannabis Patients Alliance in Denver. But like many, before she became an activist, she was a patient.

She was diagnosed with fibromyalgia in 1988. Fibromyalgia is a chronic malady, overwhelmingly striking women, and is characterized by severe pain, fatigue, digestive upset, sleep disturbance, and anxiety.

Given that Teri is now 56, she's had fibromyalgia nearly her entire adult life. She was treated with the usual progressive shopping cart of drugs – anti-inflammatories, NSAIDs, opiates, and anti-depressants.

That is, until 2009, while doing marketing for the bike taxi business she shared with her husband, Teri met the owners of a medical marijuana dispensary in her office building that she soon did work for as well.

It was an education. As she began using marijuana for her illness, she also dug deep into the broader implications and realized what a benefit it would have been for her own stepfather, dying of lung cancer a few years earlier.

"Hey, cannabis is not the 'cure all' but people need knowledge and empowerment."

Teri has both a day and night regimen. To fall asleep she smokes or vapes indica. To stay asleep she'll usually eat a brownie or other sweet. Daytime, she vapes a high CBD or sativa strain, supplemented by a muffin, cookie, or candy as needed.

As Colorado became a medical marijuana state in 2001 and a legal marijuana state in 2013, outsiders mistakenly think it's just one big happy party. Because recreational marijuana and medical marijuana offer different solutions they also require different formulations of CBDs and THC, and other cannabinoids. While children usually don't receive THC for seizures, for instance, adults don't need to be protected in the same manner. Teri says, "Don't discount the value of THC for therapy. Plus the higher CBD strains are typically low in THC."

This issue is now a business and political one, as expected, since Colorado's recreation business far surpasses its medical one, and limitations are placed on the strength of purchasable marijuana.

Thus, there is a need for the Cannabis Patients Alliance to lobby and educate on behalf of its member-patients and the population at large. Think of the patient caregivers – experts – as compounding pharmacists, customizing the patient's prescription, as opposed to shopping off the rack at "Harry's Pot Shoppe."

Colorado is also home to the country's first "Medical Marijuana Scientific Advisory Council."

Teri was appointed by the Governor as the representative for patients, the sole non-medical, non-scientific member.

She's earned her seat at the table.

Today, only **7%** of doctors would agree to write a prescription for cannabino-pathic medicine.

Chapter

3

Why pain is well, such a pain.

Pause a moment and simply think about the word "pain."

Its reach extends far wider than the skinned knee of a child, the "Excedrin" headache, the pain in the neck that travels south, becoming the figurative pain in the ass; the pain of loss; the pain of love.

Pain has evolved into a metaphor for so many things disagreeable, great and small, that it's easy to forget one of the worst pains of all: the pain of the unsolved but very real chronic illness. People with this type of pain are dealing with both the symptoms of the illness, which typically include physical pain, and the pain of hopelessness.

In the course of interviewing patients who have benefited from using medical marijuana, and listening to them recall their struggle to find help – answers and relief – with such pain, I found their recollections to resemble those of people with Post Traumatic Stress Disorder (PTSD). The pain they described is the pain of not knowing if they will ever again enjoy a normal, uneventful day. (And who but the recently ill or the plane crash survivor will enjoy and welcome a dull day?)

Many think it's therapeutic, or healthy, to talk about how they felt during the struggle to find help, how they coped, and how they reached the goal of living that normal day, having discovered the benefits of medical marijuana.

Yet, while I listened to these medical autobiographies I recall a doctor who advised me it's unhealthy to rethink trauma because the brain doesn't realize it's watching a rerun but "thinks" the experience is happening all over again. If true, that helps explain why PTSD can be just an endless loop of old pain initiating new pain.

Pain relief is big business. Transparency Market Research estimates it's a $30 billion business in the USA. And that's just the legal business. We are accustomed to relieving pain, immediately, and the industry serves that need with products for every ache. Yet, painkillers can kill more than pain. It's just so damn easy to pop a pill to solve a problem.

What are the major pain relief categories?

Non-prescription pain relievers: NSAIDS.

They are cheap.

Advil, the most popular brand of ibuprofen, costs about a nickel a tablet, give or take. So we buy them in tubs, containing 500 pills, because, hey, there's another pain just around the corner.

They are everywhere.

Medicine cabinets in every home, supermarket, chain store, even gas stations. (Naturally, driving can be a real headache.)

They are legal.

Of course, they're legal. We don't give it a second thought.

They are recommended.
By all the people we trust: Parents, doctors, friends.

But we know pills also have a dark side. Just read the 8-point type on the bottle for all the warnings:

- This product may cause stomach bleeding.
- This product may cause a severe allergic reaction including hives, swelling, shock.
- This product may increase the risk of heart attack or stroke through long term use.

They look like little candies, M&Ms without the logo, so it shouldn't be a surprise we eat them like candy.

If and when we read about the side effects, we don't think they will actually happen to us.

Then we have more than the garden variety of headache or muscle ache.

Perhaps a sports injury sustained at the gym, overdoing our resistance training. Or we take a fall on the ice. Or we're in a car accident.

We take the painkillers for weeks or months at a time. Then, poof: we develop stomach or kidney problems, and now we really need a doctor.

Ibuprofen is but one example of the cheap, convenient, universal, and legal pain relievers. Until 1984 it was actually a prescription drug in the U.S. It's a non-steroid anti-inflammatory drug, or, NSAID. Perhaps our pain didn't respond to ibuprofen so the doctor recommended something more powerful.

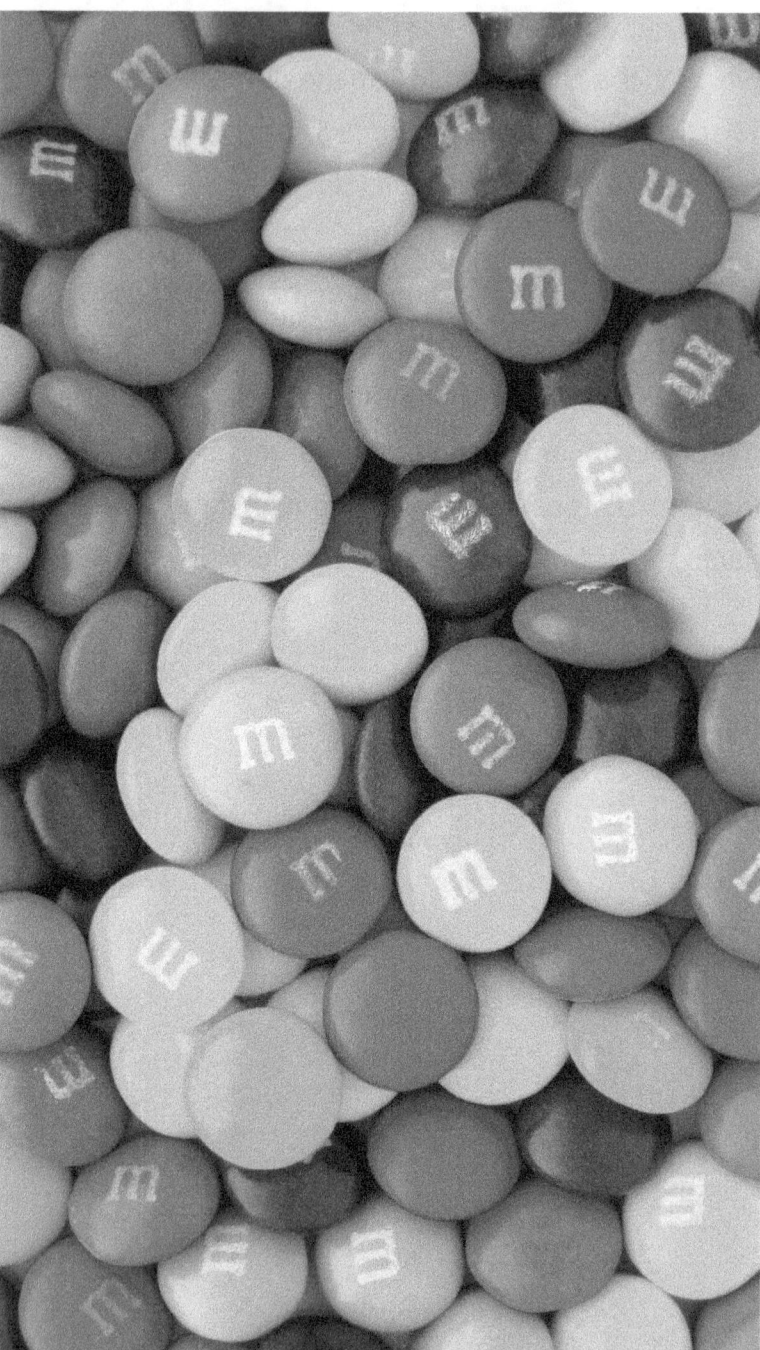

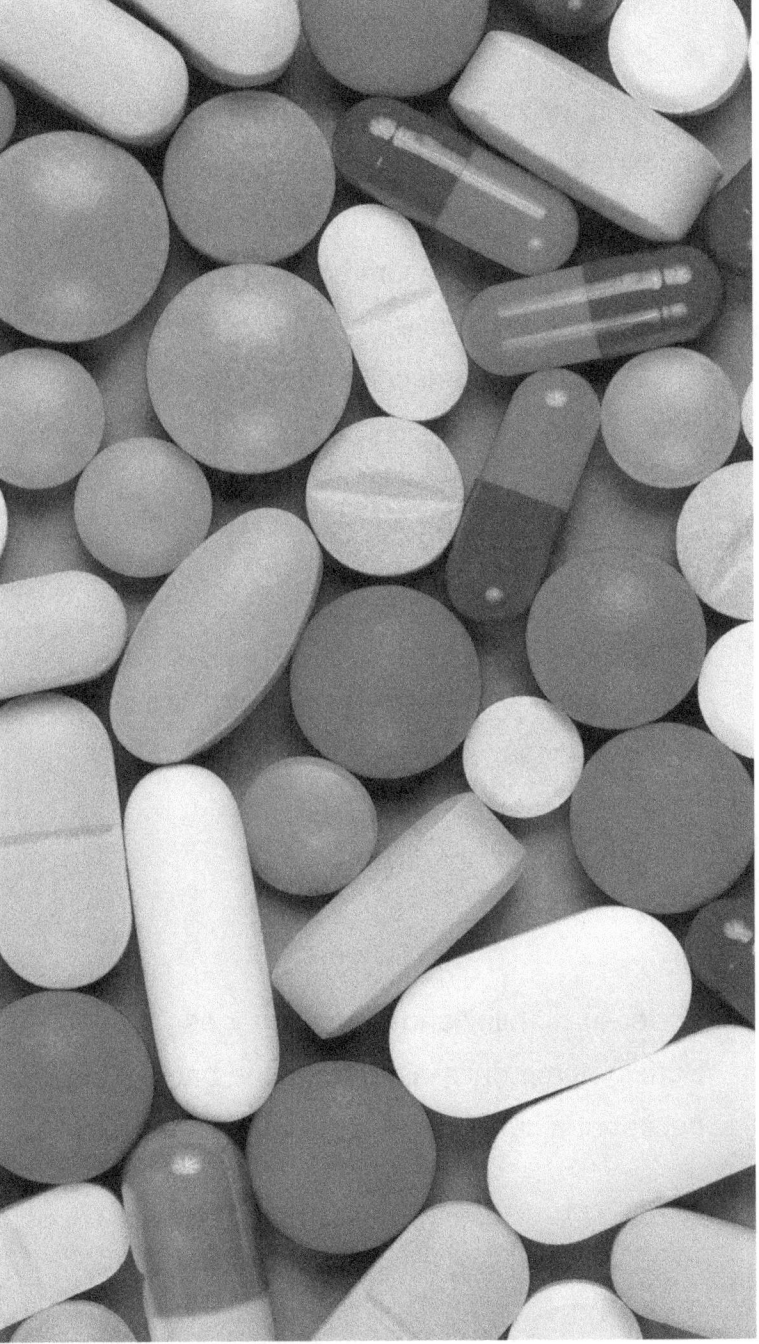

Corticosteroids

The pills on the next rung up the pain-relief ladder, corticosteroids, require a doctor's prescription because they are more powerful (and dangerous). Prednisone is the most commonly prescribed steroid for pain, but because of an all-star list of potential side effects, it's typically prescribed for a very short time (usually a week).

Side effects can include:

- Weight gain
- Headaches (let's hope you're not taking them for headaches!)
- Insomnia
- Thinning of the bones
- Acne
- Ulcers
- Hyper-excitability and mood changes
- Buffalo hump (increased fat at the back of the neck; not a cut of meat at your local steakhouse)

Opioids

Opioids even sound dangerous. They are natural or synthetic forms of opiates. And opiates, of course, are derivatives of opium. Think of them as opium's grandchildren: they may not look like their grandparents, but they have the same genes. They are used for what doctors call acute pain, meaning great pain, and are often prescribed for short-term pain after surgery. (Unfortunately, there is often long-term pain after surgery, too.)

Well-known opioids include morphine, codeine, and oxycodone. Yes, that oxycodone. The one that's infamously abused, as it can create a high similar to heroin.

Side effects or misuse of opioids include:

- Addiction
- Breathing problems
- Nausea, constipation, itching
- Death (a permanent side effect)

Oxycodone is such an attractive target for desperate thieves that many pharmacies post signs they don't even carry it.

Next stop, surgery.

When we mention surgery, we conjure all the actors and scenery:

Lying on our backs, nearly naked, except for the peek-a-boo gown. Looking up to see the green army of masks and machines. "We will see you when you wake up."

We wonder, "Will we?"

The instructions to countdown from 100, but we likely will only make it to 95.

Then, pffft, we are out like the proverbial light. And probably pray that we simply wake up, whole. Yet, Americans undergo thousands of surgical procedures each year just to relieve pain from assorted injuries and bad luck.

We overcome our fears of the surgeons and surgeries because we believe they will fix us like new, and because this slice of medicine has been ingrained in us since we were old enough to sit up and watch a hospital show on TV.

Wouldn't life be different if George Clooney played a medical marijuana doctor on TV?

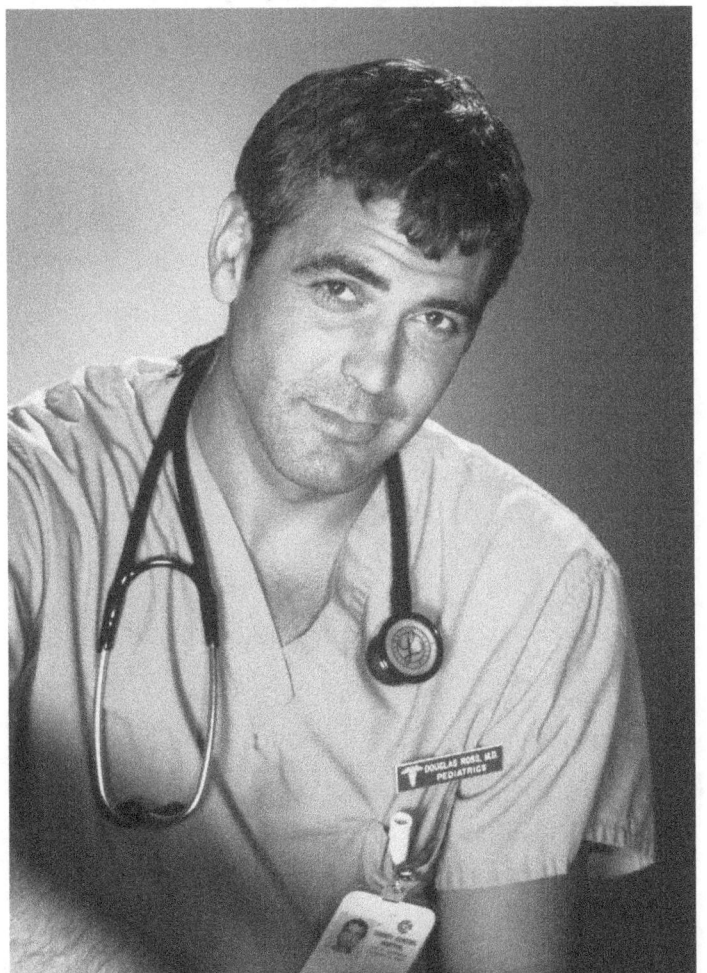

Ray Mirzabegian

Realm of Caring, Los Angeles, CA

Ray Mirzabegian, an optometry professor, was just looking for a way to reduce his daughter Emily's seizures. He didn't set out to become a medical marijuana activist.

Emily's seizures began when she was five months old. They appeared just three hours after her measles vaccination.

(According to the Centers for Disease Control, the MMR vaccine – measles, mumps, rubella – is perfectly safe for 99.9% of children. However, four children in 10,000 may experience temporary seizures. Albeit a very small number unless you're the parent of one of those four children.)

Emily was diagnosed with generalized tonic-clonic seizures. You may not know what they are.

She experienced episodes in which all of her muscles stiffened. She would let out a loud cry or scream, then lose consciousness, fall to the floor, and often bite her tongue as she turned blue. Next, her legs and arms would alternately jerk and relax. She sometimes lost bladder or bowel control. Afterwards, she slowly returned to consciousness, remaining drowsy or confused. A typical seizure would last three minutes.

Three minutes.

Imagine watching your child seize, perhaps multiple times a day.

So between that first day and the time she was eight years old, Emily tried thirteen different medication regimens until Ray waved the white flag on pharmaceuticals.

Ray reached out to Realm of Caring in Colorado Springs, Colorado. He'd heard about the success that epileptic patients had there with Charlotte's Web, the high endocannabinoidal medical marijuana without the THC-providing high.

Emily's rapid improvement prompted Ray to lobby the Stanley Brothers to permit him to open a Realm of Caring facility in California, the first outside Colorado. This facility employs a team effort between the child and family, internist, neurologist, and Realm of Caring.

What's the success rate? Ray says 70-76% of patients' seizures are either eliminated entirely or significantly reduced. And this comes after most patients first try the conventional epileptic drugs through their physicians.

As Ray reminds us, "Nothing works for everybody."

Meanwhile, when you visit the Epilepsy Foundation website the only mentions of medical marijuana appear in the section where visitors and patients post comments to each other. The Foundation has yet to take an official position.

Nothing works for everybody.

4

How Marijuana Makes us Feel Better and Be Better.

This chapter introduces the role of endocannabinoids. In order to appreciate how medical marijuana improves our health let's take a closer look. After all, you may not be qualified to teach high school biology but you will understand there is actual science at work here.

We know plants include many healing properties. It's easy to forget in a pharmacy-driven world that plants and their derivatives were the original basis of medicine. Their active ingredients continue to be studied in the present day.

We have a tendency to embrace the tools of "modern medicine" – analysis, testing, pharmaceuticals, surgery – and reject "ancient medicine" as, well, ancient. We categorize herbal medicine, that is, medicine based on the healing power of plants, as "Chinese medicine": perhaps, good enough for the Chinese but insufficient for modern Americans. But if we simply put the categories into a little box, and stick that box into a drawer somewhere, then we may be sufficiently open-minded to what actually is effective in fighting illness and its debilitating effects.

That would be real progress.

It's not just flowerpots.

Our homes are filled with beneficial plants. And I don't just mean the cucumbers and carrots in our refrigerator's vegetable drawer.

Our medicine cabinets probably have a tube of ointment whose active ingredient is **aloe vera**, which relieves the pain and distress of many burns.

The tea jar may have **chamomile**, a variety used to calm us and prepare us for sleep.

Before **henna** became the ingredient of temporary tattoos, it was used as an anti-bacterial agent.

If your black **licorice** actually contains licorice root – typically, it's a very small amount – your stomach may benefit from reduced ulcers.

Catnip doesn't just make cats happy. It relieves (human) cold symptoms and is especially helpful when breaking a fever by promoting perspiration. The foxglove plant is the source of digitalis, the drug used to prevent congestive heart failure.

Jesuit bark is the source of quinine, used to treat malaria.

The **periwinkle** plant is the source of Vinblastine, the chemotherapy drug used to treat many cancers including brain cancer.

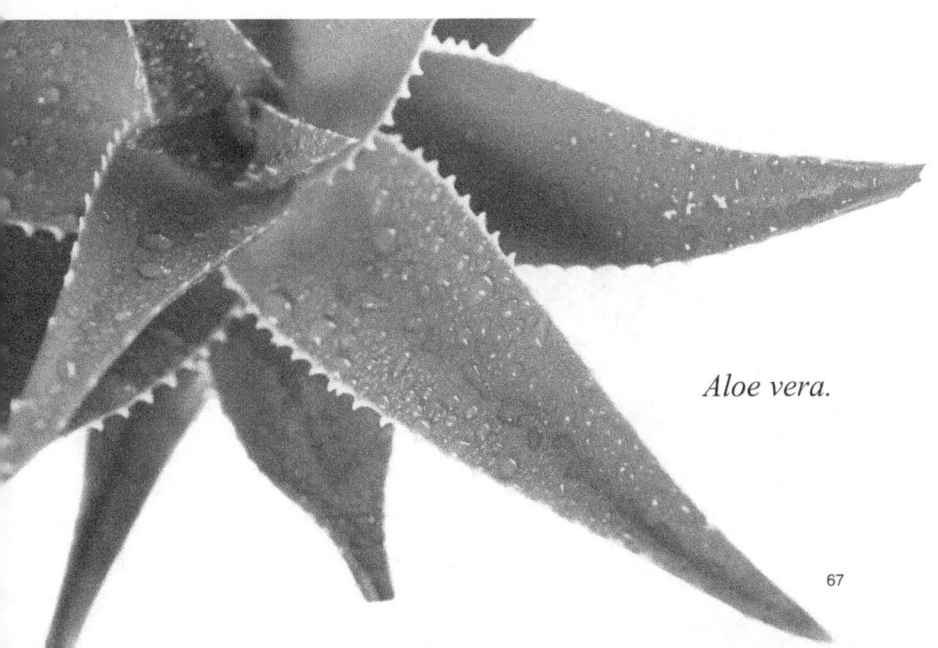

Aloe vera.

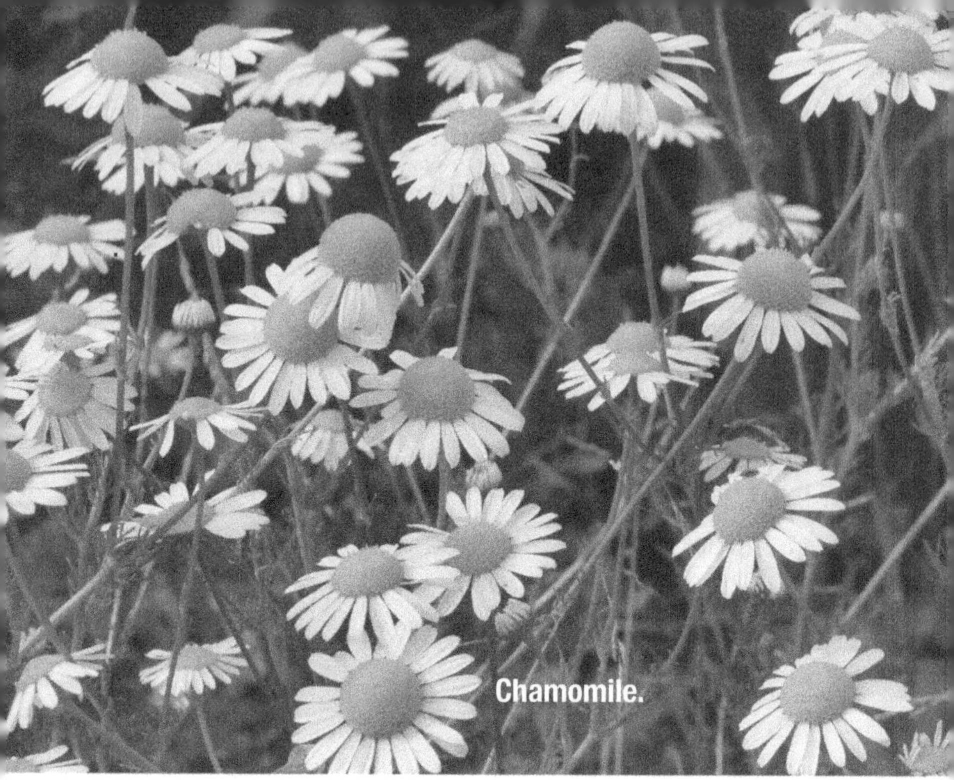

Chamomile.

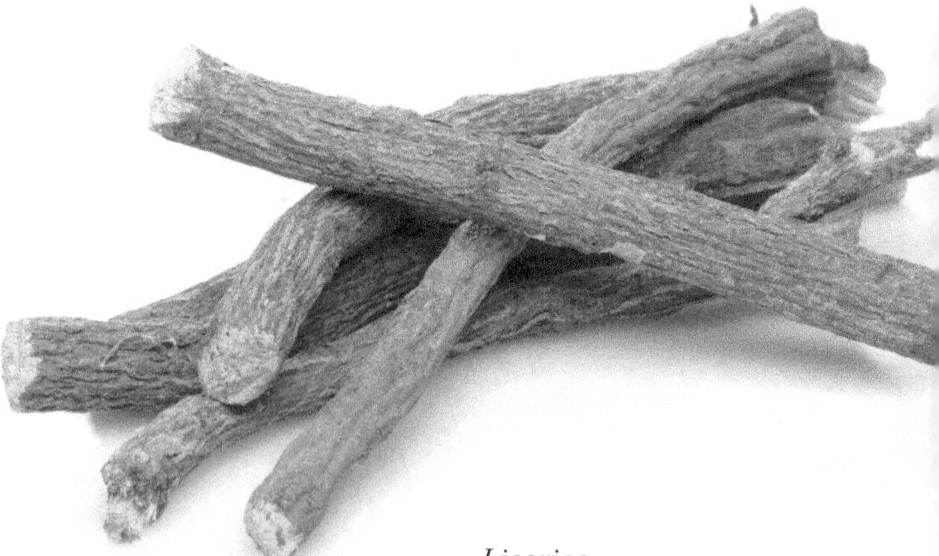

Licorice.

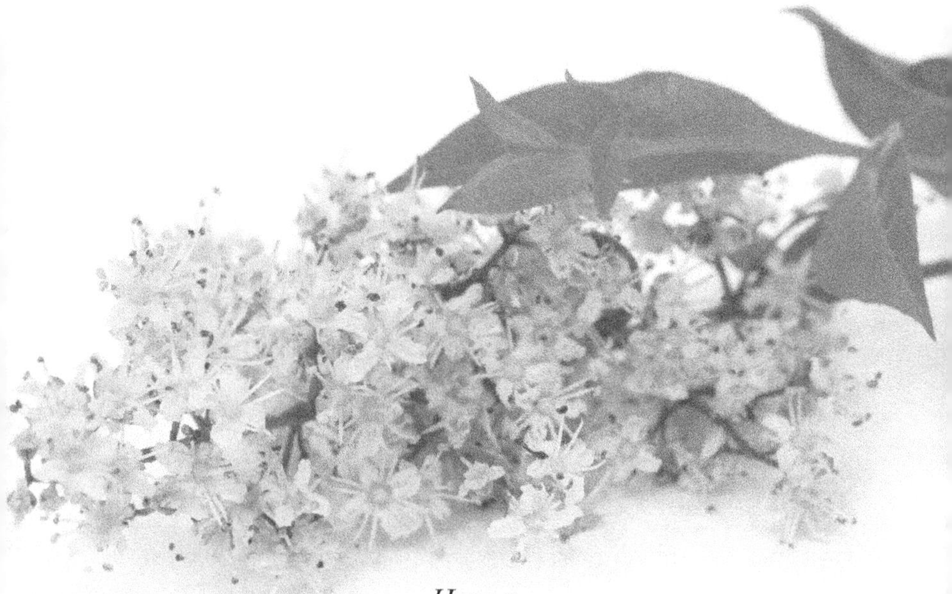

Henna.

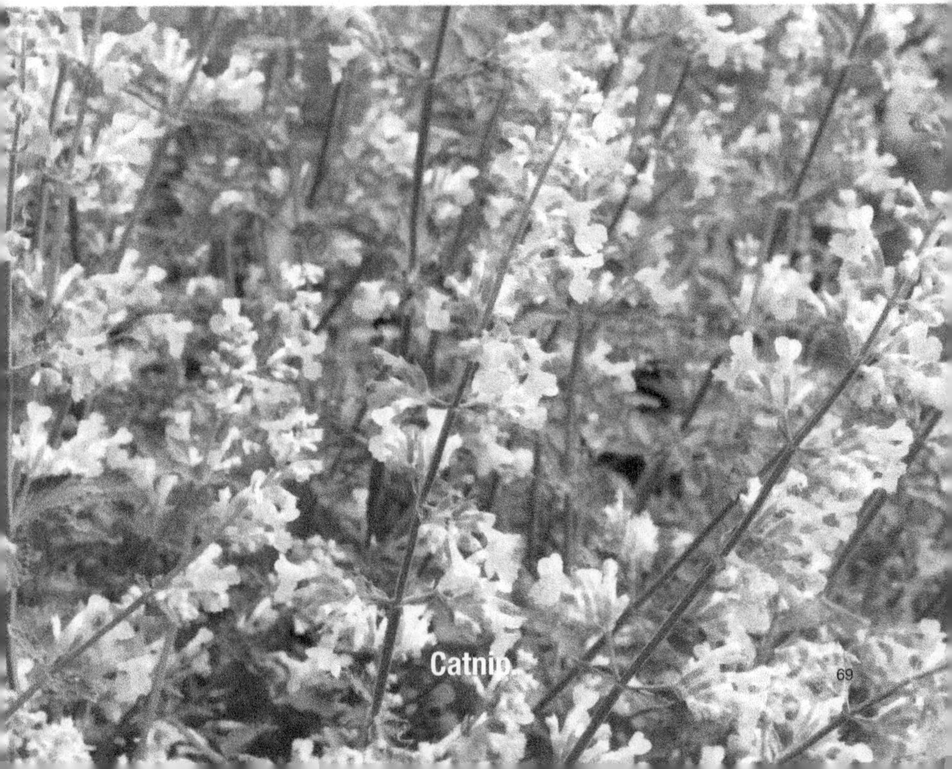

Catnip.

Marijuana chemistry.

Marijuana is a very complex plant containing dozens, if not hundreds, of naturally occurring chemical compounds. While they don't all have therapeutic or psychoactive agents, many of them do. This we know based on the limited amount of research conducted, given the legal and political restraints.

The marijuana compounds that produce any kind of healing and feeling in humans are called cannabinoids. The best-known cannabinoid is delta-9-tetrahydrocannabinol, or THC.

This is marijuana's recreational star ingredient, as it provides the high. But it also provides some of marijuana's healing elements.

Cannabidiol (CBD) is the leading compound in marijuana that promotes healing and does so without creating the psychoactive result, which makes it useful treating patients who don't want the high or patients who are children. (Refer to our earlier discussion of Charlotte's Web in Ray Mirzabegian's story.) Demand for marijuana with a high CBD content is increasing dramatically.

THC and the remaining cannabinoids that don't provide the "high" but provide the healing, all work because they travel to the body's cannabinoid receptors.

Scientists have identified more than 100 chemical receptors in the body. Among them are at least two types of cannabinoid receptors, CB1 and CB2. CB1 is located in the brain, specifically in the hippocampus and cerebral cortex, the primary locations of memory and knowledge, respectively. The receptors interact with marijuana's active compounds and produce the psychoactive effects including heightened sensory awareness, a happy state, and pain reduction.

CB2 receptors are outside the brain and are also called peripheral receptors. They are found in the immune system and certain organs, as well as in white blood cells. As you probably know, it's the white blood cells that fight disease when the body is attacked by illness.

Cannabinoid receptors convert Marijuana to Medicine.

These receptors regulate:

- Learning and memory
- Motor skills
- Pain relief
- Body temperature and heart rate

Endocannabinoids: marijuana's relatives in the body.

Left to its own devices – without the introduction of marijuana – the body produces substances that trigger the CB1 and CB2 receptors. These substances are called endocannabinoids or ECBs.

Research conducted in the early 1990s revealed cannabinoid-like neurotransmitters, the first of which was named anandamide, Sanskrit for bliss. These receptors were found in the cerebral cortex, which controls higher thinking; the hippocampus, the home of our memory; as well as the brainstem, which is the most primitive part of the brain and controls basic reflexive functions such as breathing.

The discovery led to today's research (and production) of endocannabinoids, the science behind Charlotte's Web, the medical marijuana produced by the Realm of Caring.

The ECB system plays a role in many body functions. Think of it as a corporate CEO who has many departments reporting to him including:

- Immunity
- Inflammation
- Neurotoxicity
- Blood pressure
- Appetite and gastrointestinal function
- Mood

In fact, scientists have yet to discover a single human physiological system that isn't affected or regulated by the ECBs.

This evidence makes unbiased people think if we use the ECBs in marijuana as "vitamins" to enhance the body's ECB system, especially a body function that is under stress, a person's health is likely to improve.

However, it's worth remembering there are at least another 99 chemical receptors that also play a role in physiological regulation. Neurologists don't subscribe to a single command and control structure. Instead they are likely to say, "Everything works with everything."

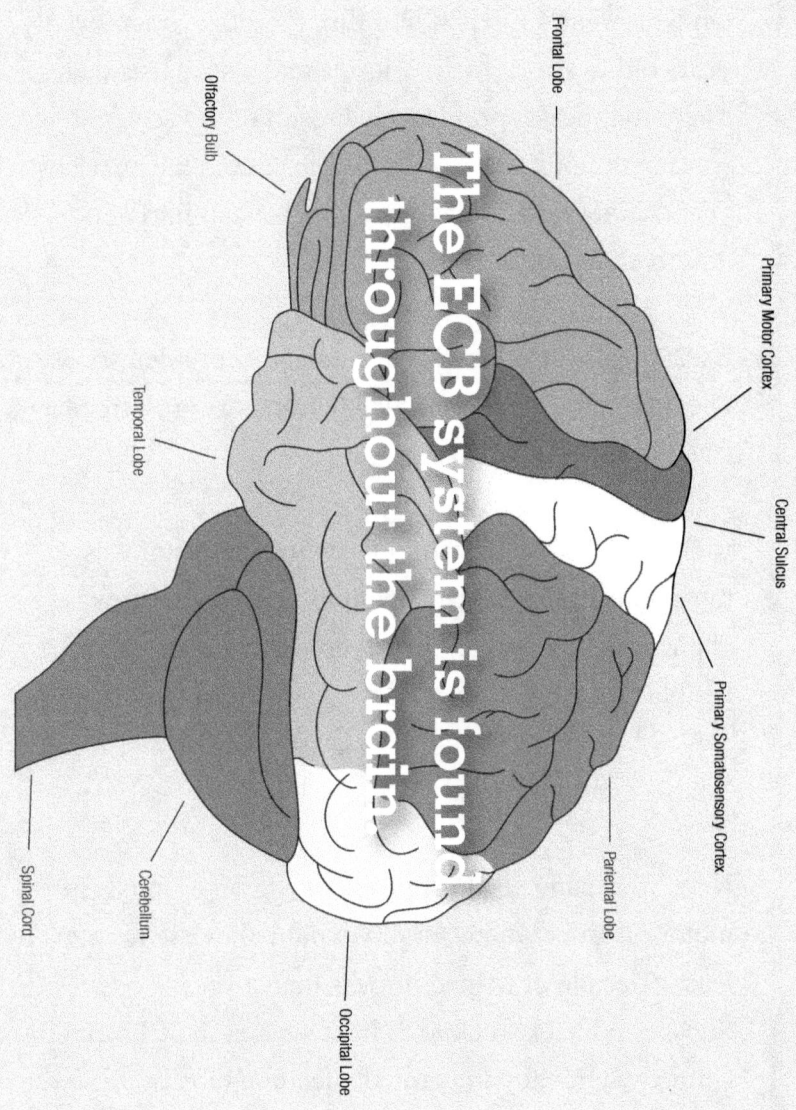

The ECB system is found throughout the brain

Frontal Lobe

Primary Motor Cortex

Central Sulcus

Primary Somatosensory Cortex

Olfactory Bulb

Temporal Lobe

Pariental Lobe

Spinal Cord

Cerebellum

Occipital Lobe

Mimi Friedman
Colorado Springs, CO

On New Year's Eve, 2002, Mimi Friedman, then twenty years old, was driving in Florida and was rear-ended. The initial health problem as a result of the accident was continuous, chronic back pain. But in the next few years her symptoms cascaded to what can fairly be described as out of control.

By 2006 she developed gastrointestinal problems, unexplained ulcers, for which her doctors prescribed a steady flow of antacids.

In 2008 she was constantly throwing up. Mimi was miserable and her doctors couldn't explain what was happening. Desperate, they even removed her gallbladder.

Yet her symptoms continued.

Next, they suggested the problem was an esophageal motor disorder which surgery would alleviate for at least a decade. It helped for less than a year.
She moved back to Ohio to be treated at the Cleveland Clinic, where they implanted a feeding tube because

Mimi was constantly dehydrated and suffering weight loss.

Did I mention she also had three abdominal surgeries? And was still vomiting.

So a doctor at the Cleveland Clinic urged her to try medical marijuana even though it was illegal. Why not? What did she have to lose? She was still on the feeding tube and it was now January 2013.

The relief was immediate.

She moved to New Mexico, a legal medical marijuana state and then to Colorado Springs, where she lives today.

Mimi has not visited a hospital in nearly two years. At the first sign of nausea she uses a vaporizer to inhale her legal 100% indica strain.

Her life has been returned to her. And she's working.

Mimi has to be the happiest Chinese food delivery person in America.

Chapter

5

Lost and Found: The Medical Marijuana Doctor.

Somewhere along this pain relief journey may be the time when your doctor asks, sotto voce, "Have you ever tried marijuana?"

If you're an upright, law-abiding citizen, this question may come as something of a shock.

If you're a desperate patient who's been through hell, just seeking a normal, pain-free day, you may wonder, "Now, you suggest it. What took so long?"

But think about it for a moment. Say you live in a state where medical marijuana is still illegal.

And while it seems a day doesn't go by where one or more state legislatures are debating medical use of this drug, there are still twenty-three states where it's completely illegal, (As change is constant visit one of the sites that tracks the progress in every state, such as http://bit.ly/1A90LKB. This is the Mother Jones site and it's updated regularly.)

So how can we expect your doctor to suggest YOU break the law and procure marijuana to relieve your illness and distress? No wonder, if he does, he does it in a whisper. And you can be sure he doesn't note it in your chart.

If he does recommend marijuana, the doctor can actually be charged with malpractice and could even have his medical license suspended. Will this actually happen? Not likely. But should he risk his reputation and livelihood? Would you?

Sadly, even in states where medical marijuana is perfectly legal, many communities, unhappy with marijuana dispensaries in their neighborhoods, create new zoning laws to remove or prevent them from spreading. And medical marijuana doctors can be harassed for practicing perfectly legal medicine.
It brings to mind the demonstrations against abortion clinics and attacks against physicians that were prevalent in the 1980s but continue in many cities and states today.

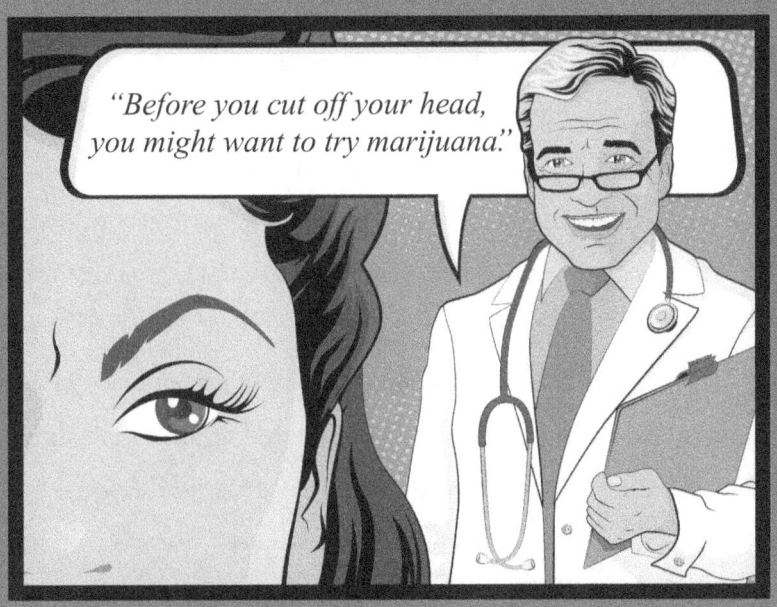

Hanya Barth, M.D.
San Francisco, CA

Hanya Barth, 69, is a child of Holocaust survivors. That experience has given her compassion and understanding for suffering of all kinds. Her goal in life has been to prevent and alleviate that suffering.

Hanya was raised in New York but spent many years living abroad. She attended medical school in Florence, Italy, together with her New York Jewish husband.

Returning to the States she first began a residency in internal medicine and then completed a family practice residency at San Francisco General Hospital. Soon, she moved to Mendocino with her seven children, living in the country and serving as the local family doc.

In 2000 she heard there was an opening in Oakland, for a cannabis doctor. Oakland was already known as "Oaksterdam," (Oakland + Amsterdam) for its liberal medical marijuana community. This prompted her to ask, "What the hell is a cannabis doctor?" Indeed.

But taking a cue from her previous experience learning new forms of treatment from the patients themselves she listened to their stories and discovered medical marijuana's "most amazing healing properties."

Hanya admits, modestly, "I have a gift for receiving patients' information and spirit." By listening with her soul as well as her stethoscope, she learned much. For example, patients suffering form Post Traumatic Stress Disorder could have various physical symptoms or be depressed, anxious, lethargic, moody, but just not know why.

Today, she directs 17 offices and 10 other doctors, while continuing to better understand and discover how to best recommend from among the myriad of strains and hybrids of medical marijuana now available. And the scientist in her welcomes the ongoing research to better understand how and why medical marijuana helps so many patients with so many ailments.

Still she acknowledges, "We are far from done."

6

History & Hysteria: How We Got Here.

We should think of plants as the original drug companies. Except without the medical-industrial complex, insurers, whopping profits, and of course, HIPAA.

Plants, including cannabis (the Latin name for the marijuana plant) preceded man, probably by tens of millions of years. There is evidence cannabis has been used as a medicine for over 5,000 years and until the 20th century actually enjoyed a good reputation.

Tombs in China reveal more than one shaman used cannabis as "recently" as 3,000 years ago. (And while they didn't attend a good American medical school they were probably very knowledgeable, especially for the time.)

Good news travels fast. Cannabis was also used in India (1400 BCE) and Egypt, including inside the tomb of Ramses II (1200 BCE). And hemp, the taller varieties of cannabis, was an exceedingly popular crop used in textiles, paper, and of course, rope.

Cannabis was one of many patent medicines in the post-Revolution U.S., which probably didn't burnish its reputation as patent medicines were neither "patented" or taken seriously as "medicines"; rather, marijuana was an ingredient in various tinctures or extracts that promised to cure, well, everything. This was likely an example of some early branding where the entrepreneurs performed the production, product naming and distribution, earning the sobriquet "snake oil" salesmen.

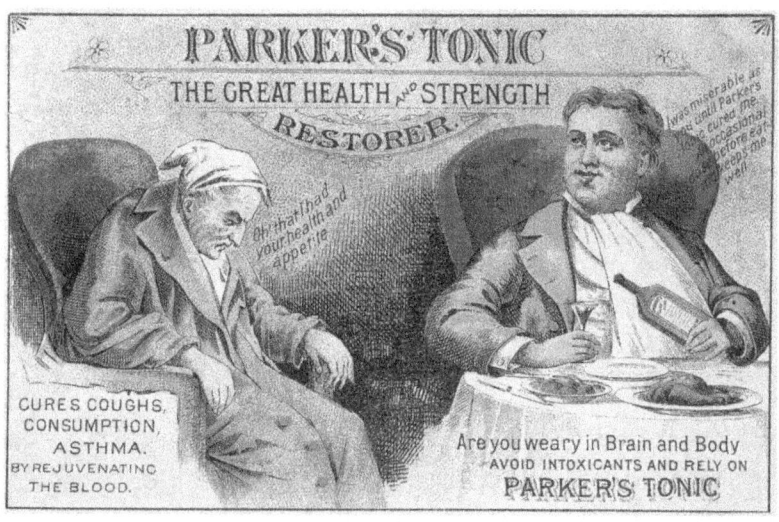

A man and a plan.

Like a character out of HBO's Boardwalk Empire, Harry J. Anslinger, practically single-handedly, criminalized marijuana in America. Anslinger, a Pennsylvania native, was the assistant prohibition commissioner at the Bureau of Prohibition.

Shortly before Repeal of the Olmstead Act, which created Prohibition in 1920, Anslinger was named the first Commissioner of the Federal Bureau of Narcotics, an arm of the U.S. Treasury Department, in 1930.

Anslinger told the story that as a child he was deeply affected by young morphine addicts in Altoona, PA, which set him on his course for life.

Marijuana was still a micro-issue. The Anslinger team grew concerned that Mexicans brought the smoking habit to the American southwest. Marijuana was also popular among jazz musicians and their followers. Jazz, of course, is an original American brand of music founded primarily by African Americans.

Anslinger used his mistrust of these two groups, Mexicans and Blacks, to successfully lobby Congress to enact a Federal law against marijuana and then to publicize it through an Anti-Marijuana radio campaign. He was convinced marijuana made people uncontrollably violent, and employed that belief as a tactic to scare the populace:

"By the tons it is coming into this country – the deadly, dreadful poison that racks and tears not only the body, but the very heart and soul of every human being who once becomes a slave to it in any of its cruel and devastating forms.... Marijuana is a short cut to the insane asylum. Smoke marijuana cigarettes for a month and what was once your brain will be nothing but a storehouse of horrid specters. It makes a murderer who kills for the love of killing out of the mildest mannered man who ever laughed at the idea that any habit could ever get him."

This is pretty strong stuff, certainly much stronger than marijuana itself. Anslinger spent much of his career defending his anti-marijuana position and attacking anyone who disagreed. This included the

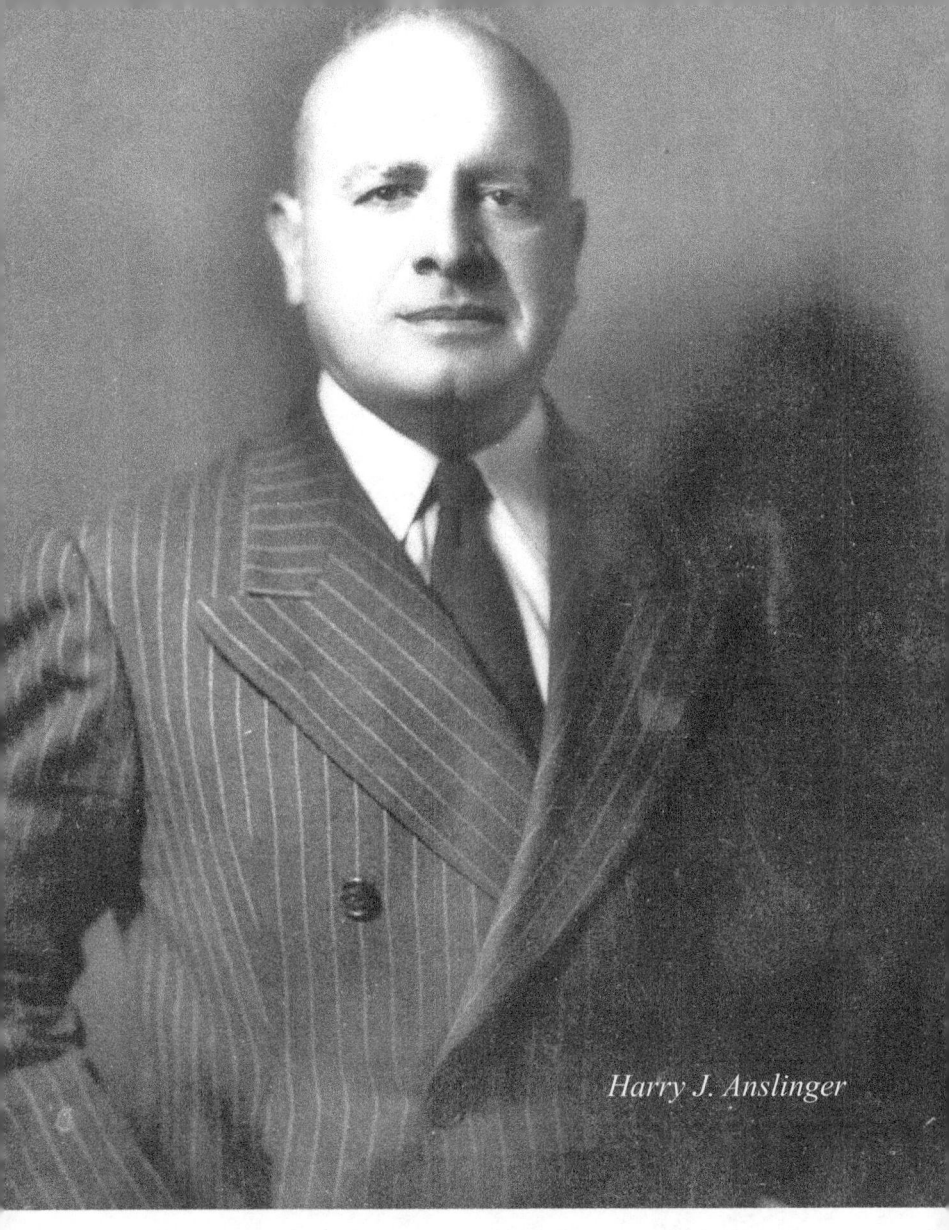

Harry J. Anslinger

1944 LaGuardia Committee Report, chaired by New York mayor, Fiorello LaGuardia, that determined marijuana smoking didn't lead to addiction.

Anslinger had a remarkable 32-year run at Narcotics, similar to J. Edgar Hoover's at the FBI; he was even reappointed by President Kennedy in 1961, before he retired the following year.

Reefer Madness.

What has been described as the "grand-daddy of all-time worst films," wasn't always such. Born as "Tell Your Children," a 1936 film created by a church group to warn parents of the danger of marijuana, Reefer Madness was soon purchased by producer Dwain Esper, and re-cut for the "exploitation" market, a broad category of low-budget propaganda films.

The plot, such as it was, revolved around an unmarried couple, Jack and Mae, as marijuana dealers, targeting high-school students, (spoiler alert!) that leads to a hit-and-run accident, manslaughter, rape, madness, and suicide; remarkably, no one gets the munchies.

Personal note: Reefer Madness was still on the propaganda trail when I attended high school in the

1960s. I vividly recall being shepherded into the auditorium with all the ninth graders for our indoctrination. Most of us in the audience took it seriously; the teachers appeared to be covering their mouths to keep their laughs inside.

It really wasn't until the 1970s when Reefer Madness became a cult favorite on college campuses, after the founder of the National Organization for the Reform of Marijuana Laws (NORML) Keith Stroup, purchased a copy and raised thousands of dollars by charging students $1.00 admission.

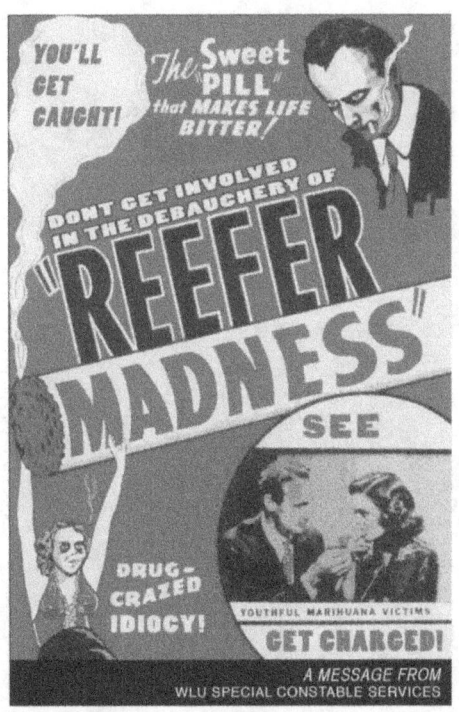

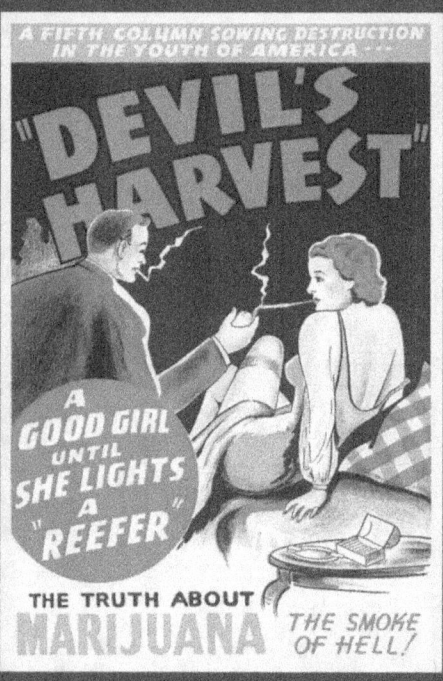

Beware! **Young and Old — People in All Walks of Life!**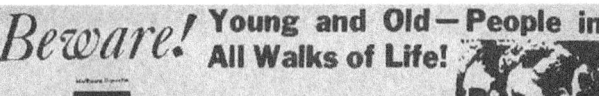

This **may be handed you**

by the friendly stranger. It contains the Killer Drug "Marihuana"-- a powerful narcotic in which lurks

Murder!   Insanity!   Death!

WARNING!

Dope peddlers are shrewd! They may put some of this drug in the 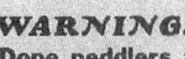 **or in the** ☕ **or in the tobacco cigarette.**

WRITE FOR DETAILED INFORMATION, ENCLOSING 12 CENTS IN POSTAGE—MAILING COST

Address: THE INTER-STATE NARCOTIC ASSOCIATION

(Incorporated not for profit.)

53 W. Jackson Blvd.   Chicago, Illinois, U. S. A.

Allison Ray Benavides

San Diego, CA

Allison is a social worker. She has three children, including a five-year-old son, Robby. In 2012, when Robby was three and a half, he suffered a grand mal seizure, "out of the blue." The neurologist prescribed the anti-epileptic drug, Keppra. It barely helped, and Robby was soon having up to 75 seizures a day.

Then they tried Depakote, but he continued to have 25 seizures a day. Every day. As Allison recalls, "When you have that many seizures, there isn't time for much else."

Unfortunately, Depakote was also unsuccessful in stopping the seizures. This was especially bad news because Allison knew that when two different medicines fail to halt the seizures, there is a 93% chance that no other medicines will work either.

Allison was already reading about medical marijuana. She joined Facebook groups where she heard about Charlotte's Web, a strain of marijuana that is heavy in cannabidiol (CBD), one of the cannabinoids, like THC, naturally found in marijuana. Charlotte's Web is the name of the grown and cultivated strain by the Stanley brothers who founded "The Realm of Caring Foundation" in Colorado. The Foundation was created to provide counseling and cannabinoid products to clients, particularly, children.

Unable to travel, Allison was fortunate to meet Ray Marzabegian. You'll recall, Ray is Emily's dad, a child with Dravet Syndrome, a rare and severe form of epilepsy. Ray had successfully treated her with Charlotte's Web and was authorized by the Stanley brothers to open a Realm of Caring location in California.

Robby became one of their first patients. The CBD-heavy marijuana given to Robby comes in the form of an orally administered oil. Six weeks after he began taking the oil, he was seizure free. He continues to take it, preventatively, once a day.

February 11, 2015 marked his one-year anniversary of being seizure free.

7

Crawling to the Present.

Richard Nixon, a man of great contradictions, opened the door to China and tried to open the door to marijuana by creating The National Commission on Marijuana and Drug Abuse. The Commission recommended the elimination of all penalties for personal use. Soon, both Oregon and Alaska decriminalized marijuana.

Then the American Medical Association, not exactly a radical organization, also endorsed decriminalization, as did the American Bar Association, the American Psychiatric Association, and the National Council of Churches. It was literally an all-star team advocating that marijuana had a bad rap and it was time to alter that perception and focus on drugs that are actually dangerous versus propaganda that was dangerous.

But the trend stalled during President Carter's administration when Lee Dogoloff replaced Dr. Peter Bourne as the White House drug advisor. Dogoloff is a prime example how one person could turn the marijuana ship around, as he saw the nation's attitudes toward decriminalization (and legalization) had become dangerously positive. He framed the discussion differently:

"We had been extremely concerned about what has been an increasing social acceptance of drug abuse in our society and we need to begin to change that."

Once again, marijuana would become the poster child of drug abuse and forced to wear the costume of a gateway drug, despite mounting evidence that the costume didn't exactly fit.

President Reagan authorized spraying Paraquat, a powerful herbicide toxic to animals and humans, and linked to Parkinson's disease, on discovered marijuana crops to discourage growers. Naturally, this created a little paranoia among marijuana smokers as they didn't know if their supply was really toxic.

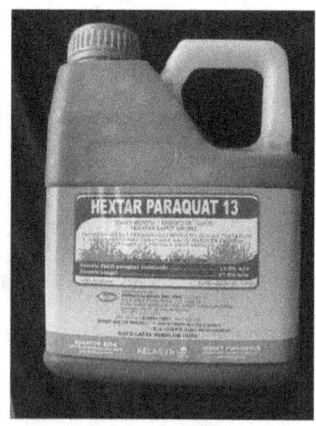

The green scare continued under President George H.W. Bush's direction. In1989, the Government initiated Operation Green Merchant, seeking identities of customers who ordered indoor plant-growing equipment.

Dr. Grinspoon – remember, he was the Optimist of 1971 – reminds us the National Institute of Drug Abuse has spent tens of millions of dollars studying, really, trying to prove the hazards of marijuana. Yet there has been no scientific basis whatsoever to prove any.

This is particularly cruel to individuals who use marijuana for medicinal purposes. This cruelty was evident during the AIDS epidemic: While the DEA was overwhelmed with requests for a disease-related exception for these patients, James Mason, head of the Public Health Service, suspended the Compassionate Investigative New Drug (IND) program saying,

"If it is perceived that the Public Health Service is going around giving marijuana to folks, there would be a perception that this stuff can't be so bad."

Grinspoon also reminded us in 1971 that, given the thousands of years of testing marijuana in the human laboratory with barely any evidence of significant toxic effects, it would be pretty unlikely that any would now reveal themselves.

A little science to the rescue.

The brain contains receptors that are stimulated by THC, the principal psychoactive element of cannabis. Marijuana researchers don't have it easy. Drug companies, doctors, and patients complain about the lengthy and expensive obstacle course the government has created, albeit to protect its citizens, to bring new drugs to market through the Food & Drug Agency (FDA).

Would drug companies even create cannabis pills for mass "consumption?"

Actually, one does. The FDA approved a synthetic form of THC called Marinol. It has been produced by

a small drug company, Unimed since 1985.
It's available only in pill form, by prescription.

Marinol is manufactured with the blessing of the
government but has limited application, availability,
and utility.

The trade-off: Marinol contains a much lower dose of
THC, about 2.5%, as compared to "street"- available
marijuana, which has 12+% of THC.

Marinol also has its critics. Because its absorption in
the body is unpredictable, for some there is no
benefit; for other users the complaint is it works too
well. Patients get "higher than expected" while trying
to stimulate appetite by reducing the nausea
associated with chemotherapy.

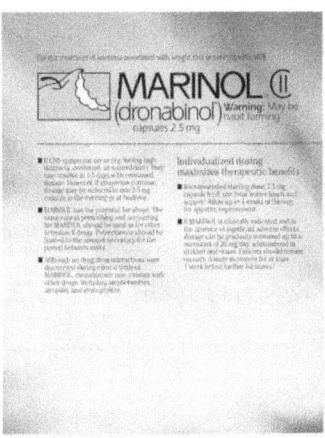

Will Marinol or its future versions come to dominate the medical marijuana market? Probably not. The drug companies can't patent a plant, which means, any company, were it legal to do so, could sell their own version. More relevant, **consumers can't manufacture their own antibiotics but they can grow their own pot.**

Marijuana's Fort Knox

Because of the federal laws against marijuana possession, cultivation, and sale, there is but a single facility the Government maintains where scientists can legally acquire marijuana. It's located at the University of Mississippi in Oxford, a property with Fort Knox-type security.

It is here, since 1968, where Mexican marijuana grows under watchful, legal eyes.

The facility is run by Mahmoud ElSohly, PhD. Its mission includes testing marijuana that law enforcement periodically rounds up, particularly from Mexico, to determine the THC levels – which are continuously rising. Researchers come here to withdraw marijuana from the only "bank" available to any studies conducted in the U.S.

Dr. ElSohly makes for the odd banker, as he's somewhat skeptical about the benefits of medical marijuana. In fact, he is a much greater believer in Marinol. ElSohly's biggest complaint about medical marijuana is the delivery system. Smoking, he points out, releases many other chemicals, not all of them friendly. Thus his work in Oxford includes finding the safest delivery system with the most efficacious results.

Which is fine, but there are few patients who won't risk ingesting those other chemicals – after all, this isn't tobacco – for the relief from hard-core pain and discomfort that overwhelms them daily.

Of course, medical marijuana doesn't have to be smoked to derive the benefits.

But isn't there a certain narrow-mindedness on the part of

the FDA that medical marijuana has to be transformed into a pill, using a synthetic formula produced by a drug company, when all along the solution is staring at us from the flowerpot?

The government was trying to appease everyone by providing a "safe" alternative to medical marijuana for the few without blessing it for the many.

Acknowledging the benefits of medical marijuana yet understanding the realpolitik of how things work in Washington – there was no chance of endorsing "real" marijuana, so they chose to do the next best thing with Marinol, by making it legal and, through grants, financially shepherding its creation at the little drug company that could, Unimed.

Then, to further enhance Marinol's prospects and reputation, the government, through the Drug Enforcement Administration (DEA), declared Marinol a Schedule II drug, the second most regulated level.

This designation raised eyebrows of practically everyone with eyebrows because marijuana, which contains some of the same compounds as Marinol, lives uncomfortably in Schedule I.

This is important because Schedule I drugs are considered the least likely to be useful for medical treatment and the most likely to be abused. Thus, marijuana is grouped with heroin, LSD, and Ecstasy, to name a few.

These drugs offer potentially severe psychological and physical dependence. Yes, that sounds like heroin. No, that doesn't sound like marijuana.

Marinol's roommates in Schedule II include methamphetamine and cocaine. Surely, even Walter White (Mr. Breaking Bad) would find this hierarchy most amusing.

Just reading through the drug Schedule below, a testimony to Henry J. Anslinger's continued influence eighty-plus years after his reign. We continue to live with a very outmoded view of marijuana.

Schedule I

Schedule I drugs, substances, or chemicals are defined as drugs with no currently accepted medical use and a high potential for abuse. Schedule I drugs are the most dangerous drugs of all the drug schedules with potentially severe psychological or physical dependence.
Some examples of Schedule I drugs are:

Heroin, lysergic acid diethylamide (LSD), marijuana (cannabis), 3,4-methylene-dioxymethamphetamine (ecstasy), methaqualone, peyote.

Schedule II

Schedule II drugs, substances, or chemicals are defined as drugs with a high potential for abuse, less abuse potential than Schedule I drugs, with use potentially leading to severe psychological or physical dependence.
These drugs are also considered dangerous.

Some examples of Schedule II drugs are:

Cocaine, methamphetamine, methadone, hydromorphone (Dilaudid), meperidine (Demerol), oxycodone (OxyContin), fentanyl, Dexedrine, Adderall, Ritalin.

Schedule III

Schedule III drugs, substances, or chemicals are defined as drugs with a moderate to low potential for physical and psychological dependence. Schedule III drugs abuse potential is less than Schedule I and Schedule II drugs but more than Schedule IV.

Some examples of Schedule III drugs are:

Combination products with less than 15 milligrams of hydrocodone per dosage unit (Vicodin), Products containing less than 90 milligrams of codeine per dosage unit (Tylenol with codeine), ketamine, anabolic steroids, testosterone.

Schedule IV

Schedule IV drugs, substances, or chemicals are defined as drugs with a low potential for abuse and low risk of dependence.

Some examples of Schedule IV drugs are:

Xanax, Soma, Darvon, Darvocet, Valium, Ativan, Talwin, Ambien.

Schedule V

Schedule V drugs, substances, or chemicals are defined as drugs with lower potential for abuse than Schedule IV and consist of preparations containing limited quantities of certain narcotics. Schedule V drugs are generally used for antidiarrheal, antitussive, and analgesic purposes.

Some examples of Schedule V drugs are:

Cough preparations with less than 200 milligrams of codeine or per 100 milliliters (Robitussin AC), Lomotil, Motofen, Lyrica, Parepectolin.

"Every
generation
lives with the
decisions of
dead men."

-- Anonymous

Lou Rubin
San Diego, CA

Lou Rubin is a successful attorney, a civil litigator, specializing in workmen's compensation cases. But in 2000 he was diagnosed with Parkinson's disease.

Parkinson's attacks the nervous system, progressively and inexorably, typically starting as a hand tremor and then moving on to tics, loss of balance, rigidity, a masked facial expression and other motor dysfunctions. There's a generalized slowness, which can progress to episodes of "freezing."

There is no cure for Parkinson's. Neurologists typically prescribe dopamine agonists to "trick" the brain into thinking it is receiving dopamine, as many of the brain cells that produce dopamine are not functioning in Parkinson's.

Unfortunately, this medicine doesn't always work; when it does, a patient will require ever-increasing dosages and experience a host of side effects, including severe nausea, vomiting, and dyskinesias, the uncontrolled body movements.

Lou, now 64, began using medical marijuana five years ago. He learned that marijuana increases the flow of messages to the brain, reducing his body's uncontrolled movements. This was a huge breakthrough. He can smoke or vape it, take it sublingually, or eat Cheeba Chews, a chocolate taffy, high in CBD.

Yet, even in California it can be difficult to acquire medical marijuana, as dispensaries frequently open and close when jurisdictions pass laws to keep them away. "It's a conservative county. The dispensaries come and go."

Lou's son Andrew is a filmmaker who has helped his Dad deal with Parkinson's and engaged with the Parkinson's community. In 2013, Andrew directed, *Ride With Larry*, a documentary about Larry Smith, a 20-year Parkinson's patient who has used medical marijuana to overcome the illness and pedal 300 miles across South Dakota. Meanwhile, there isn't a single mention of medical marijuana on the official site of the Parkinson's Disease Foundation (pdf.org).

8

How to Choose.

Fifty years ago in America, before marijuana evolved to become medical marijuana, it was still, famously, a recreational drug. It was much more dangerous in the legal sense, as many people actually went to jail for possession or distribution. Since 1970, nearly 15 million Americans have been arrested for marijuana crimes.

Yet marijuana itself, was much more innocuous. Back in the 1960s, the THC content of most marijuana was around 3%, while today's strains are usually between 10% and 15%, meaning today's marijuana potency is up to five times that of fifty years ago.

But marijuana had an outlaw legend, instilled by the government and propagated by Hollywood. Think Midnight Express, the Alan Parker film starring Brad Davis as a first-time smuggler (hashish, actually) caught leaving Istanbul to spend a very unpleasant five years in a Turkish prison.

Then there was *Easy Rider*, the 1969 countercultural film directed by Dennis Hopper, starring himself, Peter Fonda, and a newbie named Jack Nicholson. Their

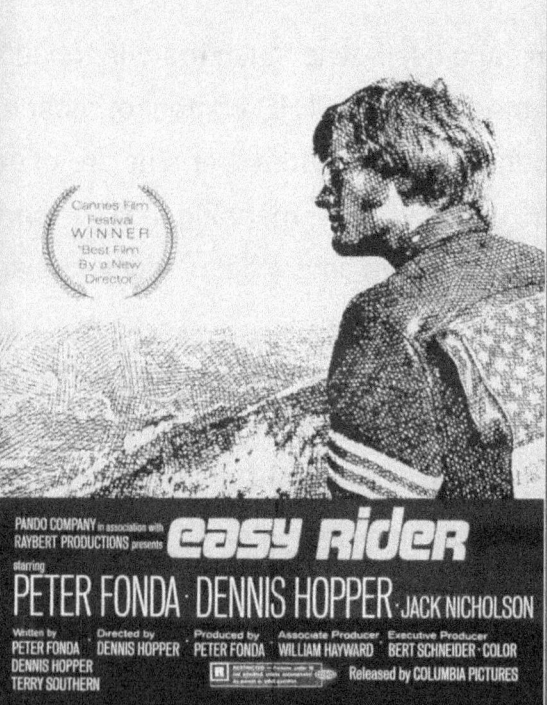

hit-the-road lifestyle, including many scenes smoking marijuana, and "bad" attitude, led to their downfall.

What these and dozens of other films had in common: no actors were seen smoking marijuana to ward off the effects of nausea.

No one talked about sativa or indica, either, just good pot.

Sativa and Indica and everything in between.

Cannabis strains are either pure indica, pure sativa, or hybrids. Marijuana growers have become very sophisticated in their botany and nearly always know that what they are planting will yield a marijuana with a particular profile.

The two dominant types are indica and sativa. While there is far from universal agreement among scientists and doctors regarding the specific effects of each, marketing-types would disagree, and claim there is enough evidence particularly among marijuana users and connoisseurs that each strain offers different benefits.

This is hardly a Coke versus Pepsi debate. Each has its following. Perhaps, given more research in the future it will be settled scientifically. Until then, consider the current nomenclature a pretty good system.

Indica.

Unless you're a grower, distributor or a member of the DEA, you're not likely to bump into a live plant. Indica is shorter than sativa making it more practical for indoor growing, but indica can still reach three feet.

The branches are close together and the leaves are wider. Indica offers a forest-like smell of pine, earth, and a touch of skunk. (But just a touch.)

Indica also boasts a higher concentration of THC, often double that of sativa.

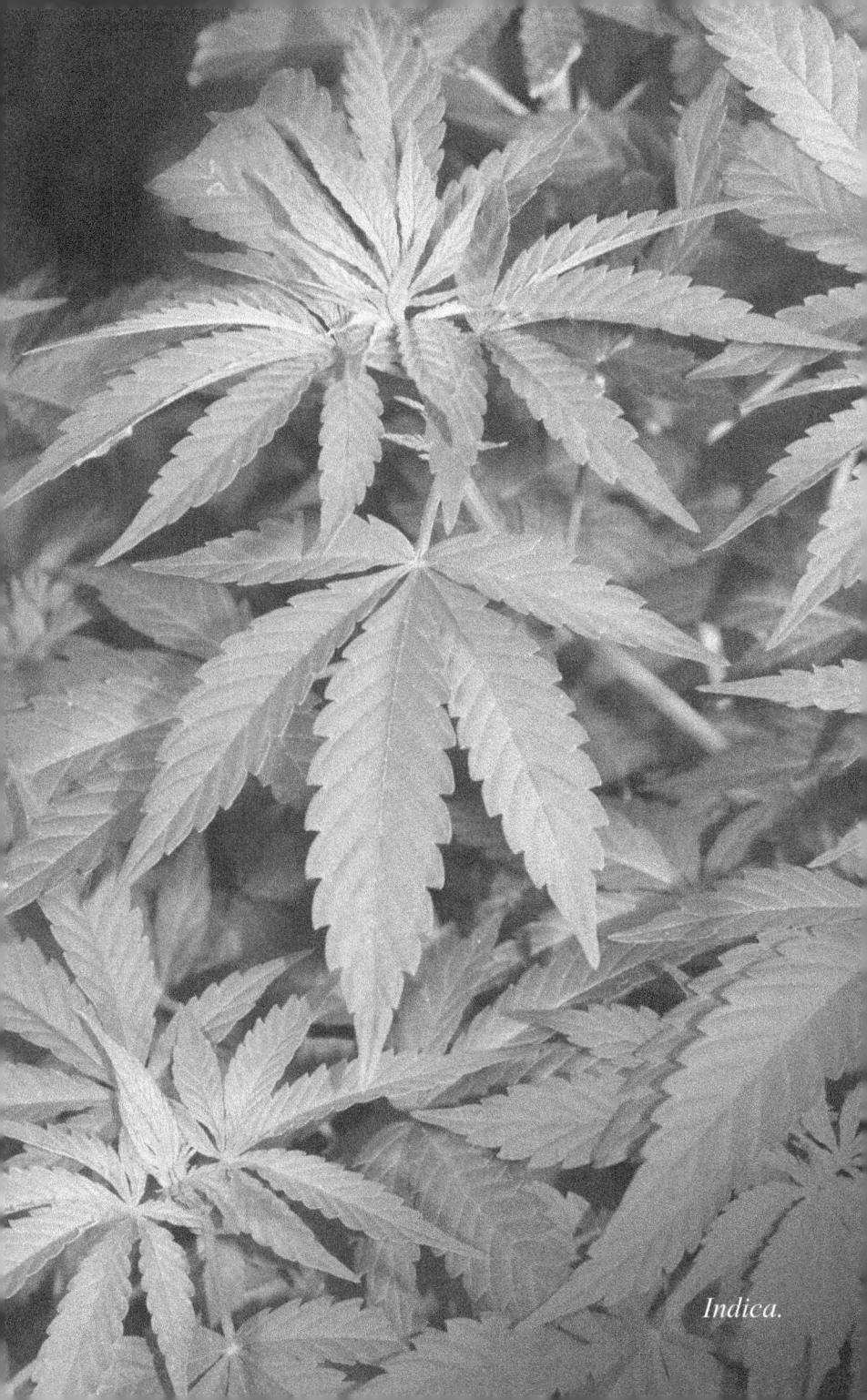

Indica.

Indica = Body

Indica is typically the medical marijuana choice for calming the body, and making sleep more likely, so it is best used at night. It is also the better inflammatory to treat pain, both local and full body.

Indica is recommended for treating anxiety, nausea, and insomnia, and stimulates the appetite.

Patients with multiple sclerosis, fibromyalgia, and Parkinson's report marked symptom reduction through use of indica. Obviously, not every patient enjoys this success, but a significant majority does. Dr. Grinspoon estimates 75% of patients find relief.

No medication offers universal relief. Even aspirin, the closest drug to a universal medicine, isn't effective or appropriate for everyone.

Indica = Body

Sativa.

Sativa plants are tall, often reaching a height of twenty feet. The branches are less dense than those of Indica. The flowers are longer and narrower.

Sativa = Mind

Also nose. Sativa plants are known to be very pungent, smelling sweet and fruity. Some say sativa strains can smell like diesel fuel, not a useful attribute, unless you work at an Exxon station.

The effects of sativa are typically energizing and uplifting. People report both heightened creativity and thinking. Sativa is also considered the choice of the daytime user.

Sativa is used to treat anxiety, stress, depression, and attention deficit disorders (ADHD). Some patients report it can be very helpful in making their brains focus.

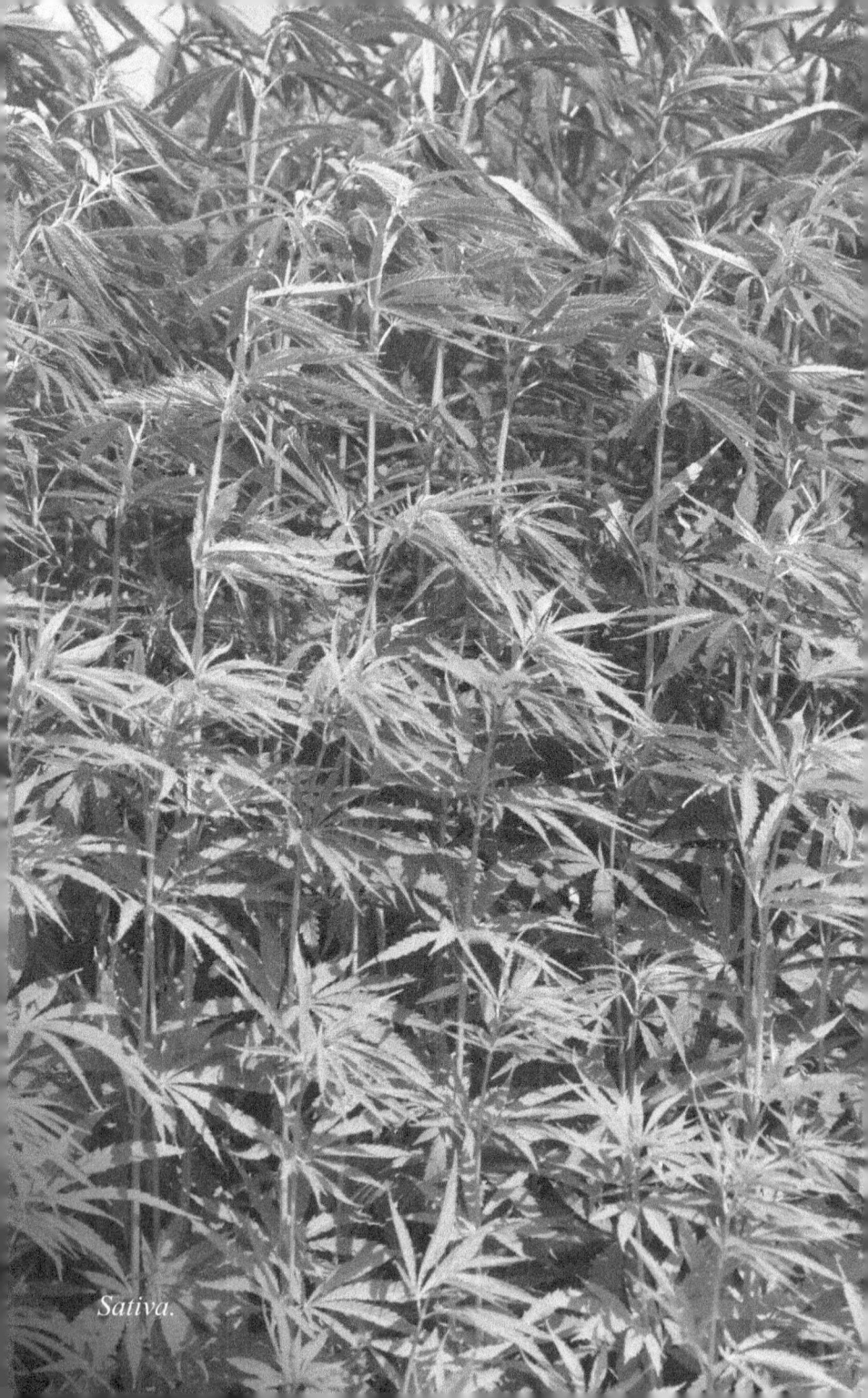

Sativa.

Hybrids.

Surely, this won't come as a surprise: There is an entire range of hybrids, each with a profile combining some of the personality of indica and sativa. The three popular categories:

Sativa-dominant hybrids.
They offer a thinking man's high, but also relax the body.

50/50 hybrids.
These claim to offer a true balance between mind and body effects. (Though the claim strongly reminds us of Miller Lite advertising claims. ("Great taste. Less filling.")

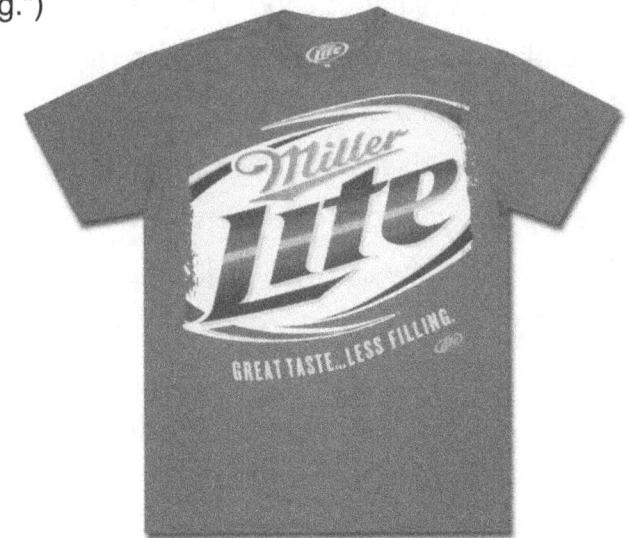

Indica-dominant hybrids.

The indica hybrids are said to offer total body pain relief plus a happy head. They can be used both at nighttime to go to sleep and daytime to relieve pain. Frankly, this group sounds the least credible, given the stark differences – indica's couch-lock and sativa's da Vinci properties – particularly if you subscribe to the entire classification system to start.

While indica and sativa are the best-known types of marijuana, they also aren't the only ones.

Ruderalis.

This sounds like a plumber's tool. The name actually refers to a plant that is the first to arrive after a major disturbance such as a drought or a fire. Believed to originally be from Russia, this thick, clustered plant looks like a place your grammar school friend will hide behind, then, as you walk by, he will jump out and shout, "Boo!"

Ruderalis have a low THC content relative to indica

and sativa, so are rarely grown for recreational use. Its use as a medicine has very little research to support it.

We understand your choices among the varieties and the hybrids are probably confusing, particularly given the overlapping benefits of each strain. We suggest you:

- Talk to friends or members of your support group to learn from their experiences.

- Talk to your doctor (if he or she supports the use of cannabis), as he or she may have learned from other patients which strain is the most effective for your situation.

- Talk to your dispensary. While the owner probably didn't go to pharmacy school, his experience with his customers is likely very helpful.

- Visit sites like leafly.com that offer reviews and comparisons.

Amy Goldman
Huntington, NY

Amy Goldman is a mom. And while she's also a wife and a big deal corporate attorney she has spent the past two decades trying to do her absolute best to be a good mom. She hasn't had it easy. Her husband is also disabled with MS.

Amy has two adult children, Elizabeth and Michael. (I have changed the names of everyone in this family for reasons that will become apparent.)

Elizabeth, the older sister, began demonstrating very odd behavior about the age of eleven. One winter day she decided she was actually a wolf and tried to sleep outdoors. Back indoors, she preferred to get on the floor, and eat out of a bowl. It wasn't long before Liz was administered anti-psychotics.

But this story isn't about Elizabeth; it's about Michael. Michael was about nine years old when his sister imploded. Early on, he was precocious and anxious, demonstrating bipolar symptoms and what doctors suggested was a proprioceptive disorder: an inability to know where you are in physical space. Certainly sounds disorienting. He researched his sister's illness. He was even administered anti-psychotic meds as a "preventative." He suffered school anxiety and soon, acute sleep disorder.

Amy: "I was miserable and wanted us all to die." The family moved upstate so Elizabeth could attend a special school. Uprooted, Michael barely attended his school as he was sleeping less than an hour a night. (This wasn't self-reported but observed.) After taking him to sleep specialists, Amy was informed they couldn't help Michael because he didn't sleep enough. Duh.

The family returned to Long Island. Michael didn't attend school, but studied at home. His teenage years ticked by: thirteen, fourteen, fifteen. Of course the psychiatrists tried the usual potpourri of drugs to get him to sleep: Ambien, Trazodone, Seroquel, but all were unable to reduce his anxiety sufficiently to earn a legitimate night of sleep.

That is, until a friend asked if Michael had tried marijuana. Amy, living in New York, and a lawyer, no less, didn't have a lot of contacts with the marijuana underworld. So she called her cousin's wife, Jody, who did. Soon, Amy was in the apartment of Bob, "the nice drug dealer in the sketchy neighborhood," and he was explaining to her the virtues of cannabis indica.

That night, Michael, then sixteen, smoked his first joint. And he enjoyed six hours sleep. Six hours! Soon, his days were better, too, as he became less uncomfortable in his own skin.

Amy: "Everything just started getting better."

Michael enrolled at Nassau Community College, spending what would have been his eleventh grade of high school. He smoked the nighttime joint, every night, to get to sleep. And usually once a day, to keep him focused. Michael became well enough to go to college transferring to a school in Seattle, where he is today, studying Economics.

"Did I get an hour of sleep most nights? Maybe not even that."

Michael Goldman

Seattle, WA

I caught up with Michael Goldman on a day off from college classes near Seattle. He was on his way to take a hike with his girlfriend in the Cascade Mountains.

Michael, now twenty-one, still Amy Goldman's son, spent his teenage years too-awake, largely seeking a good night's sleep. Now, he expects to graduate in spring 2015.

As he says, the Pacific Northwest has a very permissive attitude about people: "They let you alone. It's not just that Washington is a legal marijuana state. it's a stay-off-your-case state."You could say I can be a very anxious person, in fact, a whole new category of anxiety."

Unsurprisingly, Michael remembers things a little differently than his Mom.

He recalls an incredibly unhappy ten-year old version of himself. "Did I get an hour of sleep most nights? I don't think even that. I don't remember the days as I remember the nights. Just very depressed. Just trying to fall asleep."

"I didn't even get enough sleep for the sleep study. They kicked me out. I was twelve years old."

After exhausting the sleep pharmacy, his doctor suggested marijuana, saying they ran out of options.

Michael remembers smoking the first joint with his Mom in the room. Awkward, and it had no effect. By the fourth time he recalls lying there feeling tired as opposed to his usual exhausted self. Yet, pfft: Eight hours sleep. Hallelujah! That was five years ago. He's smoked pretty much every day since. And is living a pretty normal life. The anxiety is under control. Not all the time, but most of the time.

Looking ahead, perhaps to law school.

"Surprisingly, the ABA (American Bar Association) is against drug tests for lawyers. If they ask drug use questions, I don't want to be in the room."

Chapter

9

How to Use.

You're ready to make the leap.

Even if you've never tried marijuana, either recreationally or medically, you probably have a sense of some of the available ways to ingest it. Fortunately, there is now an ever-growing variety of choices to meet patients' needs and personal choices.

This means if you're not comfortable putting a lit object in your mouth and inhaling deeply, then don't. You're not a character on a Fox TV show going through an initiation. Rather, you're a person in pain, mental or physical, and relief with marijuana doesn't require walking across hot coals.

Smoking.

"First, do no harm." Whether this expression actually appears in the Hippocratic Oath (many believe it's actually from the Hippocratic Corpus; same Hippocrates, different document), but what matters is the meaning:

Let's not create a new problem trying to solve an old problem.

If you're uncomfortable smoking marijuana then don't do it. But don't avoid it because you think it's unsafe. It is safe.

The only connection between tobacco smoking and marijuana smoking is the smoking part.

While smoking any substance can create carcinogens, the very limited studies comparing the two have been inconsistent and inconclusive. However, if you consider just a consumption comparison it should make you feel more comfortable.

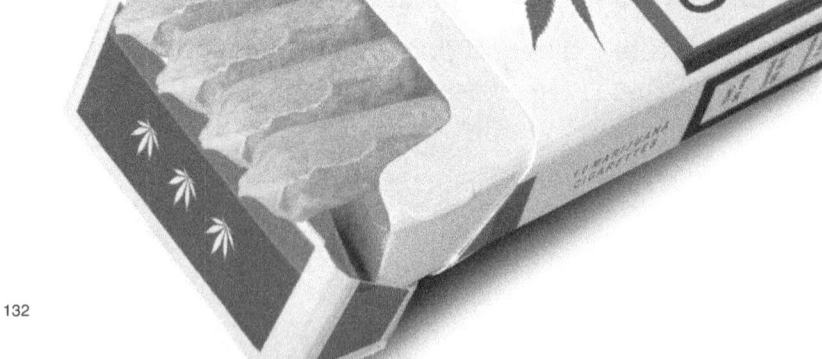

A marijuana smoker will typically take just a few puffs and be done. Sometimes, just one or two total.

A cigarette smoker will usually take a dozen drags on a cigarette.

A marijuana smoker may have just one or even two smoking occasions in a day. That would lead to five or six puffs.

A cigarette smoker will likely smoke an entire pack (or more). A pack's puffs would be about 240 in a day.

A cigarette smoker may inhale an ounce of tobacco a day.

A marijuana smoker probably won't inhale an ounce in two or three or four weeks. Even people who smoke once a day, everyday, probably smoke only an eighth of an ounce every two weeks.

While marijuana cigarettes are convenient, you are still "smoking" paper and the joint continues to burn between puffs.

Pipes.

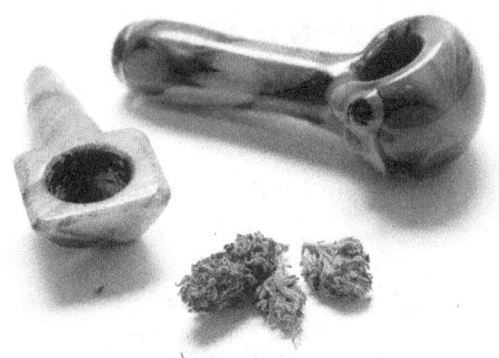

Alternatively, a pipe can be preferable for both its efficiency and economy. It only burns while you inhale and you therefore use less marijuana, too.

Pipes are inexpensive and easy to use. Simply place a small amount in the bowl, light it, and inhale deeply, holding your breath for 30 seconds. It's also a good idea to cover the pipe bowl with your hand, cutting off the oxygen, which stops the marijuana from further burning. (Just think of it as taking your foot off the gas when you want to extend your gas mileage.)

Pipe varieties also extend to water pipes. Here the marijuana travels through water (even iced water) both cooling the smoke before it enters your lungs and filtering out many of the smoke's less friendly particles.

Vaporizing.

Many patients prefer vaporizing or vaping marijuana as opposed to smoking marijuana because vaporizing doesn't require combustion. Rather, it converts the marijuana into a cool gas at a lower temperature than burning, thus eliminating nearly all the smoke and potential carcinogens.

Actually, cannabinoids begin to vaporize at about 100 degrees lower than smoking: 285 versus 390 F. Vaporizing still provides a very quick effect and enables the user to strictly control the amount he inhales.

It is the same technology that some tobacco smokers are turning to with E cigarettes. Imagine a time in the not-so-distant future you will be able to purchase marijuana fitted precisely for your E cigarette.

Until then there are vapor pens, the size of fountain pens and also significantly larger devices, not meant to be portable. (Note: the pens typically work with marijuana wax or oil.) They are in the $100 neighborhood.

Extractions

Before imagining you're in a dental chair for a painful procedure, from which you will emerge one tooth short, this isn't it.

Marijuana extractions are simply a concentrate or tincture, the latter being a liquid resulting from combining alcohol with a marijuana plant. (Actually, it's a tad more complicated, but that's the gist.)

Alcohol extractions are typically dosed sublingually, placed under the tongue with an eyedropper, for fast absorption. Sometimes they are applied directly on the skin.

Children are often given a THC-free oil in order to receive the benefits to their endobannabinoid system without the high.

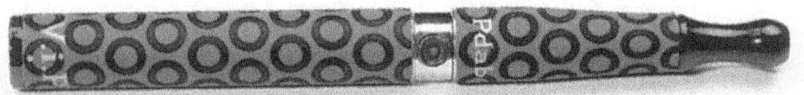

Vaporizer Pen.

Wax

An increasingly popular form of concentrate is marijuana wax. The wax is used in vaporizers but can be vaporized, too. The wax, also known as Butane Hash Oil (BHO), is formed by introducing butane gas into marijuana, producing a very potent and waxy substance. (This is definitely not recommended for DIY chemists, as working with butane can actually be quite dangerous.)

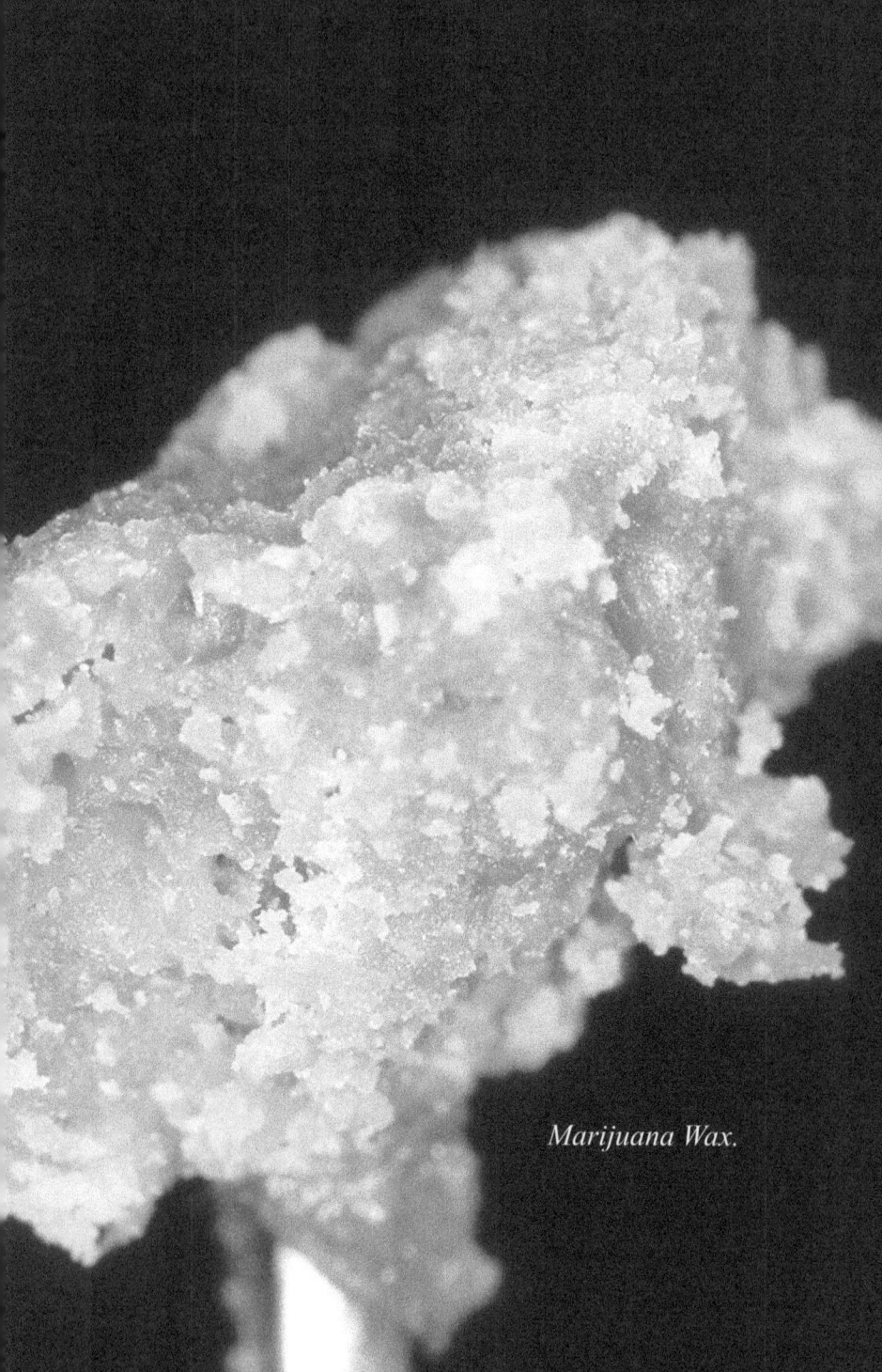

Marijuana Wax.

Edibles

As we are a nation of eaters it's hardly surprising that marijuana edibles have become increasingly popular. Recipes abound – there are even marijuana cookbooks. Eating marijuana is very different from smoking marijuana. It takes considerably longer to feel the effects so often people mistakenly eat too much, too quickly, and ultimately become uncomfortable or zonked out. Famous case: Maureen Dowd, New York Times columnist, traveled to Colorado to report on marijuana legalization. In her hotel room she consumed an entire candy bar, reporting:

> But then I felt a scary shudder go through my body and brain. I barely made it from the desk to the bed, where I lay curled up in a hallucinatory state for the next eight hours. I was thirsty but couldn't move to get water. Or even turn off the lights. I was panting and paranoid, sure that when the room-service waiter knocked and I didn't answer, he'd call the police and have me arrested for being unable to handle my candy.

While it's easy to chuckle at Dowd's naiveté and lack of experience, it's better to learn from her experience, particularly when addressing your inexperience.

A simple rule is if you purchase ready to eat cookies, candies, brownies, beverages, etc., that you ingest a small amount of that product until you can gauge the effects.

As each manufacturer uses different recipes and processes it's also prudent to try new products, carefully, as a candy is not a candy is not a candy.

Critically important: like any medicine or drug, keep out of reach of children.

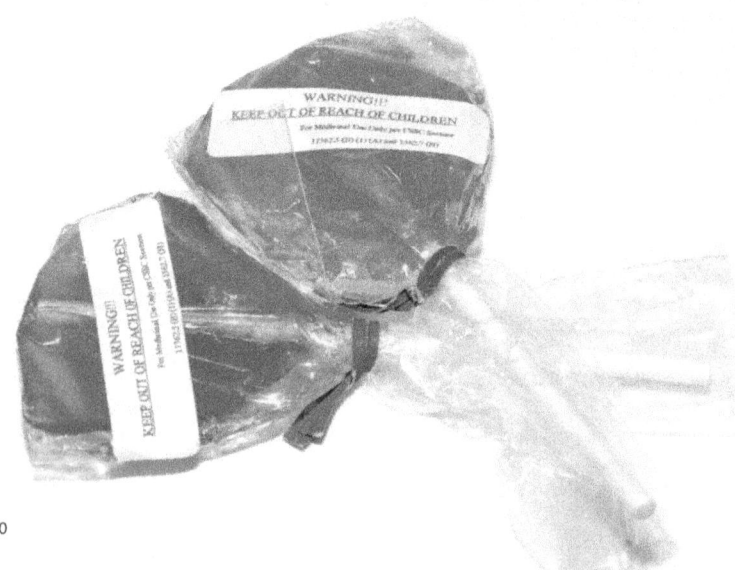

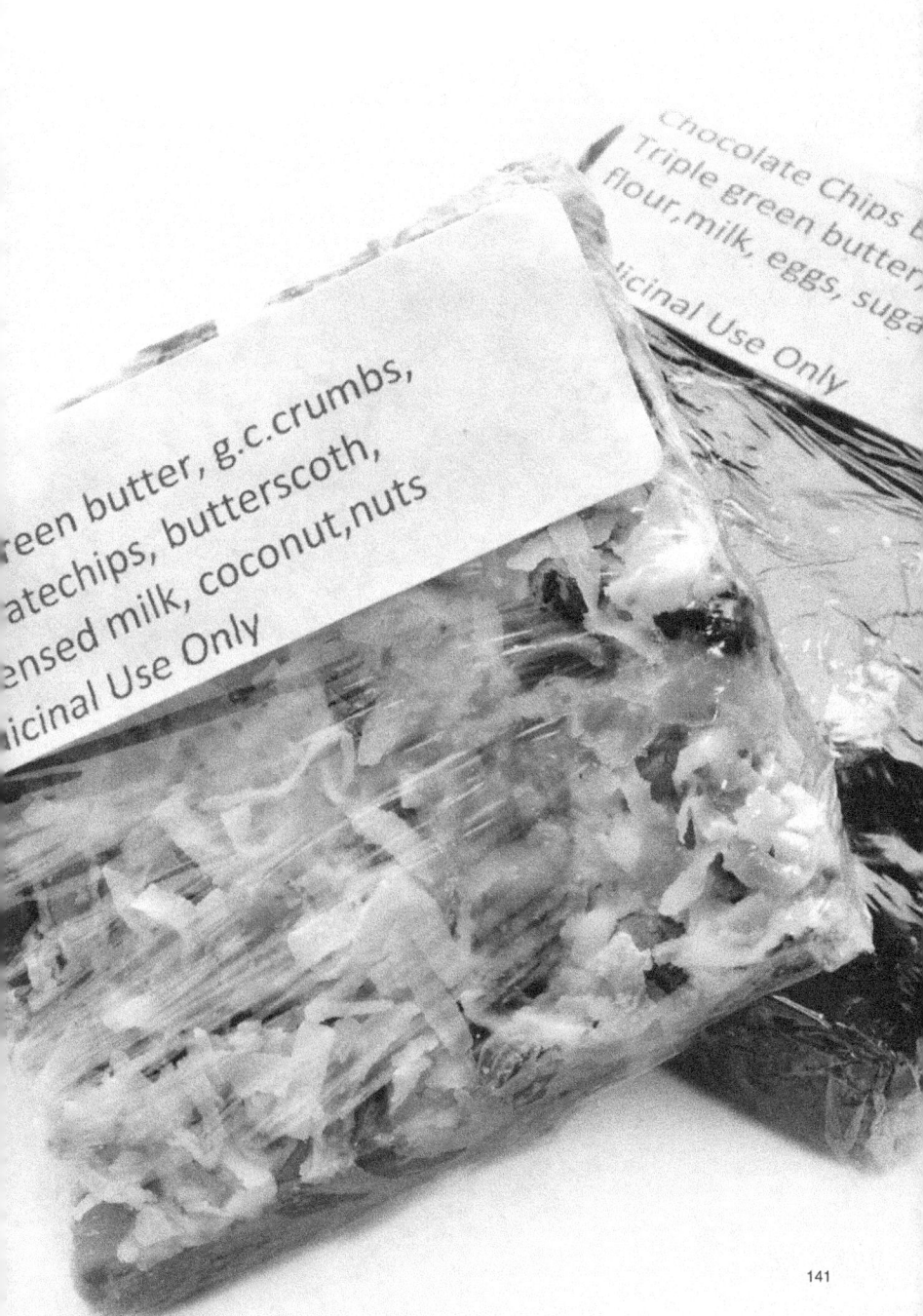

…reen butter, g.c.crumbs,
…atechips, butterscoth,
…ensed milk, coconut,nuts
…icinal Use Only

Chocolate Chips b…
Triple green butter,…
flour, milk, eggs, suga…

…icinal Use Only

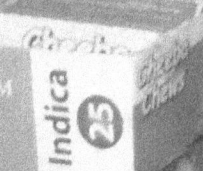

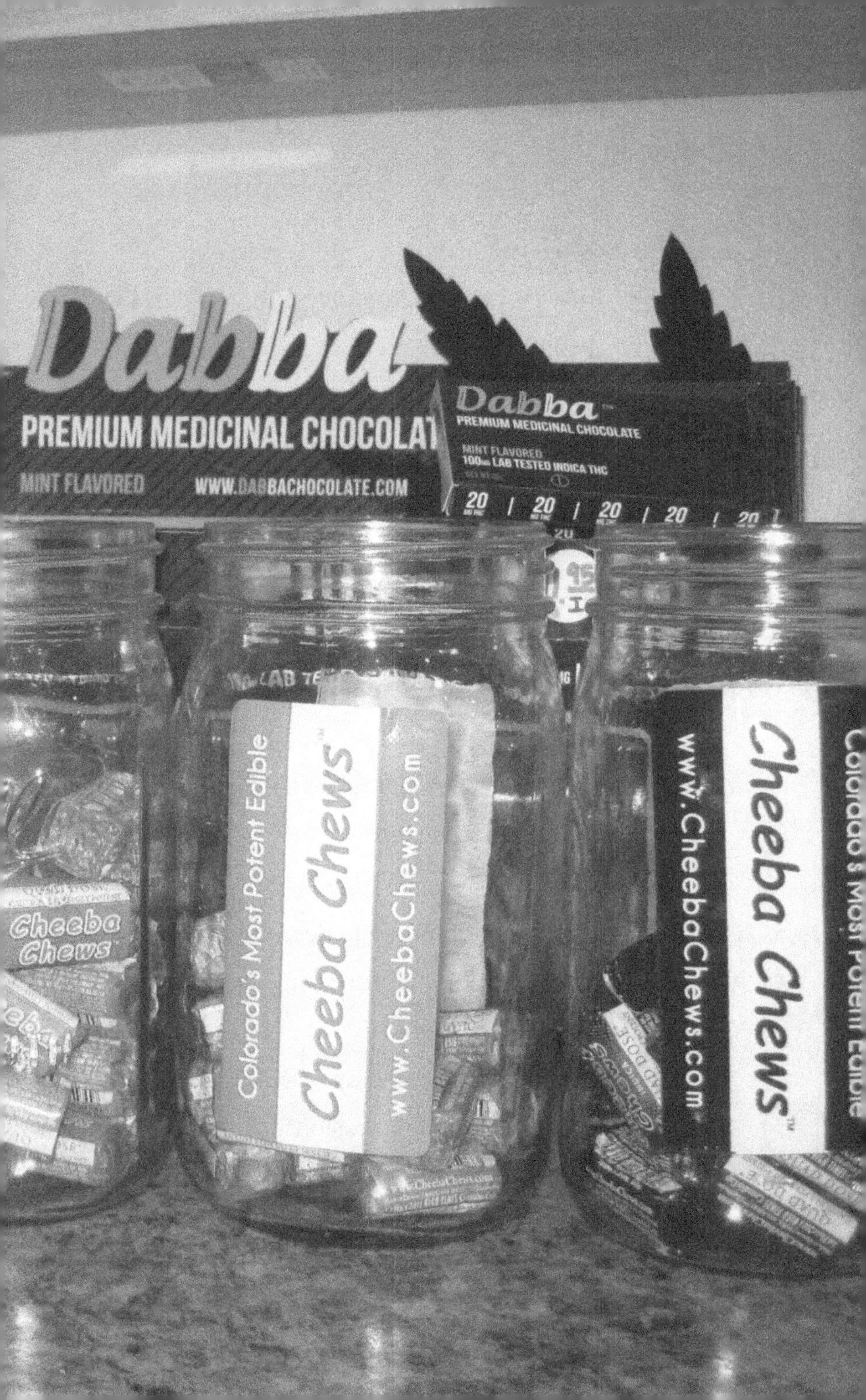
Dabba
PREMIUM MEDICINAL CHOCOLAT
MINT FLAVORED
WWW.DABBACHOCOLATE.COM
Dabba
PREMIUM MEDICINAL CHOCOLATE
MINT FLAVORED
100mg LAB TESTED INDICA THC
20
20
20
20
Cheeba Chews
Colorado's Most Potent Edible
Cheeba Chews™
www.CheebaChews.com
www.CheebaChews.com
Cheeba Chews™
Colorado's Most Potent Edible

Larry Bogart, MD
Denver, CO

Larry's story doesn't arrive in a pretty package. However, what makes the story compelling is that Larry (not his real name) has been a doctor and a patient.

Larry grew up in New Jersey, wanting to be a doctor from the age of ten. He recognizes it's been an odyssey: he attended college at Tulane; medical schools in Bologna, Italy, and Guadalajara, Mexico; then a diagnostic radiology residency in New Hampshire.

'I was something of a savant in radiology, just when mammography was becoming its own subspecialty. Colleagues said I was the best."

Larry's genetics left him prone to depression and irritability. There was bipolar illness in his family. He crashed in the mid-1990s. Drugs didn't help so he turned to electroconvulsive therapy (ECT). He twice had to tell me he had 75 ECT sessions just to make sure I heard it right. "My brain had reached its limits."

Larry lost his health, his medical license, and really, his identity. Yet he still managed to marry and have two children. In 2007 he became a medical marijuana doctor and patient, which brought him a degree of normalcy, a place where he could function again. He joined a medical marijuana practice, helped steer Denver patients through the paperwork, and provided guidance to patients seeking medicine.

"Tell me about your problem," he would say. Not everyone wanted to.

The medical licensing board of Colorado has determined Larry cannot practice while he possesses an active medical cannabis registration for chronic pain and bipolar illness.

"It's ironic: the 'approved' meds don't work for my illness, yet they are perfectly acceptable to the state." No longer married but still an active father, Larry is trying to get his license back. He reminds me he didn't lose it because of any suggestions of malpractice; he lost it because he admitted to using medical marijuana.

The cannabis, yoga, exercise, and good sleep control his pain and manage his bipolar illness. Yet he also uses legal meds on an as-needed basis, as pain, bi-polar disorder and depression are very tough opponents.

"The state has told me I can no longer practice. But they can't tell me I'm not a doctor," he told me.

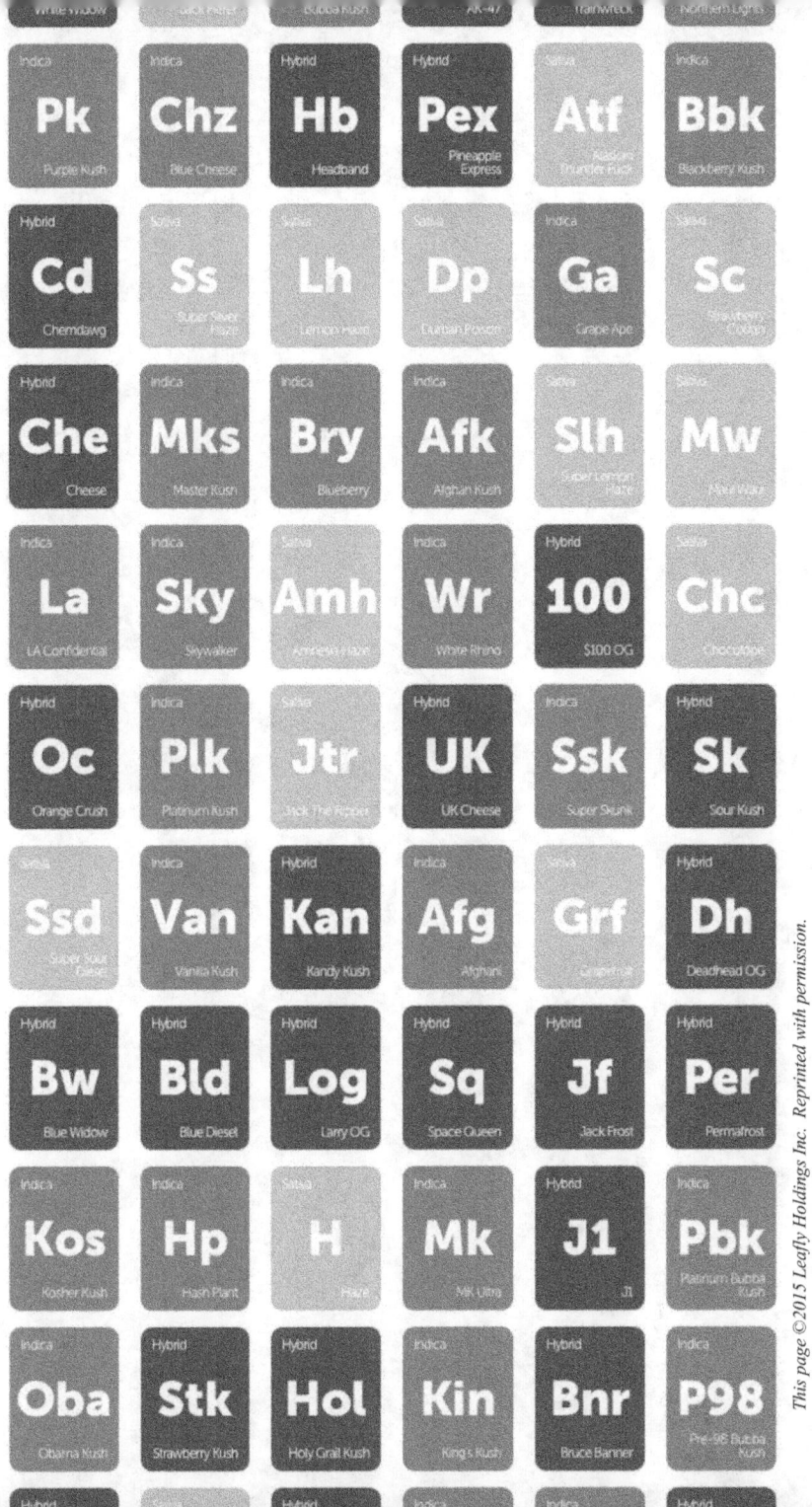

Inc. Reprinted with permission.

10

Do Marijuana Brands Matter?

Sooner or later you will be able to go to Whole Foods or CVS or, let's invent a new chain store, MariWanna, and select from a copious selection of extracts, smokes, and edibles based on your particular taste and preferred brand. Just as you now do for beer or ice cream.

Maybe the products will be under lock and key, or secured in an adult-only area to prevent children from shopping for them. Or maybe there will be free standing stores, like wine and liquor shops today. Or maybe it will be nothing like that.

Maybe Congress will gift the business to tobacco companies. Let's hope not. Yet some fear this is a real possibility given Tobacco's undying influence. (Never count the bad guys out.)

And perhaps the drug companies are waiting in the wings, despite consumers' ability to grow their own. The allure of a pill in a bottle dispensed by a person in a white coat remains very compelling.

Finally, don't forget Kraft Foods or Kellogg's or

Pillsbury. It's not so far-fetched that down the road, Corporate America will want a slice of the marijuana pie. They have the money, the distribution, and the marketing power to make their brands successful.

But let's not get ahead of ourselves. Today, there are growers, dispensaries, and marketing firms already laying the groundwork and ringing the cash registers.

(Literally, there are cash registers, as banks and credit card companies will not participate in medical marijuana commerce due to existing federal laws and fear of new laws.)

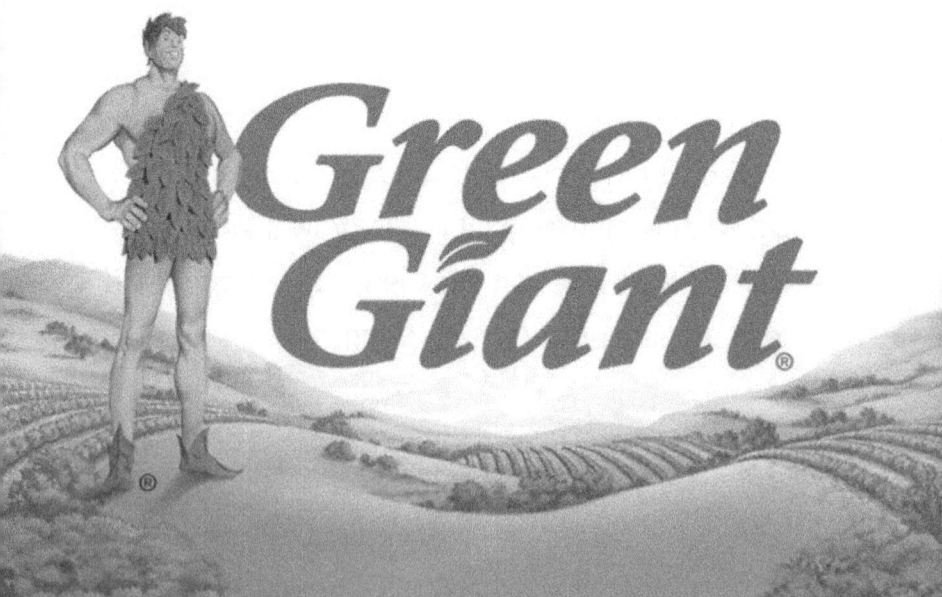

In the background are the investors, promoters, matchmakers, and other carnival characters, gathering in anticipation of a modern Gold Rush or what people are already referring to as the "Green Rush."

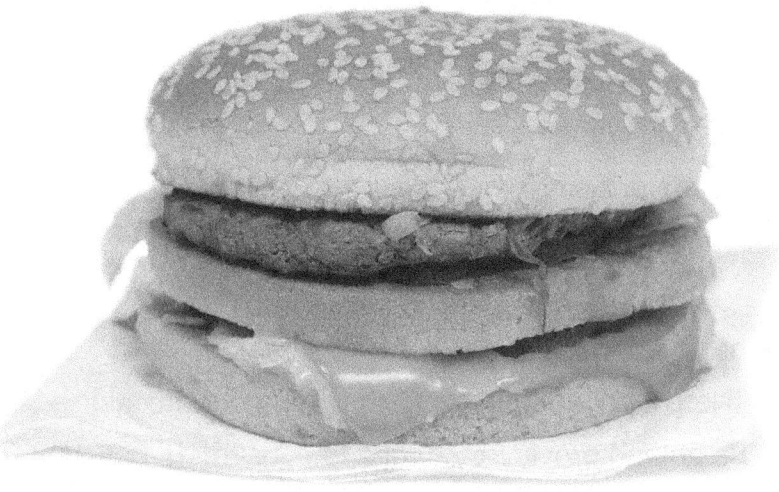

This may not be as bad as I'm making it sound. The current growers are trying to marry doing good with doing well. Many want to provide to their customers a reliable product whose properties are consistent over time, the very definition of a McDonald's Big Mac, can of Pepsi, or a hybrid strain of marijuana. All promise to deliver certain benefits without surprises or disappointments.

The brands also don't want to go broke doing it; that's the doing well part. As more states either sanction medical marijuana usage or legalize it altogether, more players will enter the business and the "business" will not be immune to economics.

There will be increased competition that should
- drive up quality
- reduce prices
- increase choice

We can imagine a day where Consumer Reports – or a similarly conventional product testing organization – will be able to provide guidance to consumers based on testable and repeatable criteria.

In the meantime growers, dispensaries, and marketers utilize rudimentary branding techniques to inspire loyalty. For instance, perhaps they create a hybrid strain that offers both the energy of sativa with the couch-slam of indica. They give it a name like "Little Red Caboose."

Perhaps, over time, that name proves uninspiring,

and it fizzles. Little Red Caboose is renamed
Chocolate Licorice. (Maybe there's a hint of
chocolate, maybe not.)

Then poof: it becomes a big success through word of
nose. It's the same formula, just different branding.

Marijuana names cannot be protected through
trademarks, though the U.S. Patent and Trademark
Office as recently as 2010 approved a few, but
belatedly realized it's actually illegal to trademark illegal products, and quickly rescinded the rule.

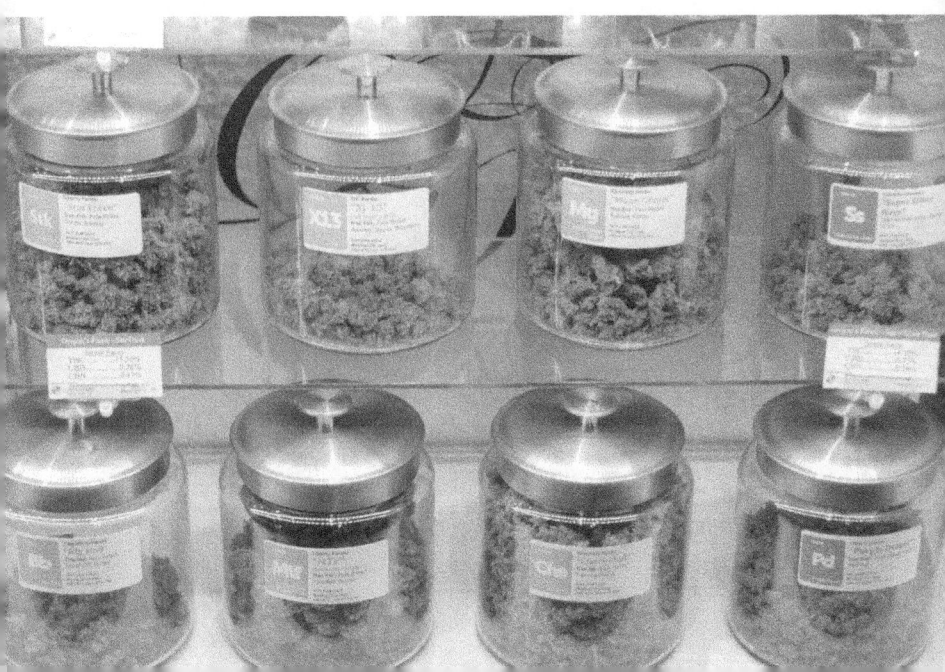

However, this doesn't stop anyone from engaging in Do It Yourself Branding. Some of the rules they use:

Flavors:
Strawberry is particularly popular. There isn't a big demand for banana.

Celebrity:
Runs the gamut from Charlie Sheen to Dr. Sanjay Gupta, the CNN medical reporter who is a medical marijuana advocate.

Heritage:
Kush and Che harken back to earlier strains.

Random:
It's well known that much of the naming is conducted during product testing sessions.

Coming from a marketing background it's easy, perhaps too easy, to be cynical about marijuana marketing. There are organizations that serve as Yelp-like review sites or clearinghouses of information about the latest marijuana brands, including detailed customer reviews. Some even include the parentage of a new brand, very reminiscent of thoroughbred horses.

Leafly (leafly.com), based in Seattle, describes itself as the world's largest cannabis community. Created in 2010 by three software engineers, Leafly is a crowd-sourced review site boasting over 100,000 product reviews.

Leafly serves both the casual and medical customer, with reviews of over 1,000 different strains. CEO Cy Scott, agrees the number of strains strain credulity, and the likelihood of "similars and sames" is pretty high.

Plus, once a brand becomes popular it isn't unheard of for other brands to just co-opt the name for their product, as well. This Cy guesses is what happened recently when the "Girl Scout Cookies" strain became very popular in California, and was suddenly available in dispensaries statewide.

Leafly has a smart-looking classification system

employing a variation of the periodic table of the elements you may recognize from high school chemistry class. It includes an abbreviation for each brand as well as effects and flavors notes, worthy of *The Wine Spectator*. Leafly also created a free app for iPhone, iPad, and Android, offering a search tool to find doctors and dispensaries, in addition to product reviews.

The intersection of branding and science begins in the laboratory. "Since there is no FDA for cannabis, the labs play a crucial role for the dispensaries and consumers, seeking legitimacy and trust," according to Scott Cathcart, Chief Strategy Officer at Steep Hill Halent in San Francisco. Steep Hill is the most mentioned facility when it comes to cannabis testing. They provide the science backbone to organizations like Leafly.

Steep Hill's trademarked product, "Strain Fingerprint" analyzes a dozen cannabinoids and terpinoids. After employing cluster analysis, they then create an attractive graphic of the average chemical makeup of each strain tested. (Cluster analysis is a statistical method that groups similar objects.)

The makeup provides confirmation to the growers that they have achieved a certain balance or objective in the strain. Then it's up to the branders to communicate the "formula" with a catchy name.

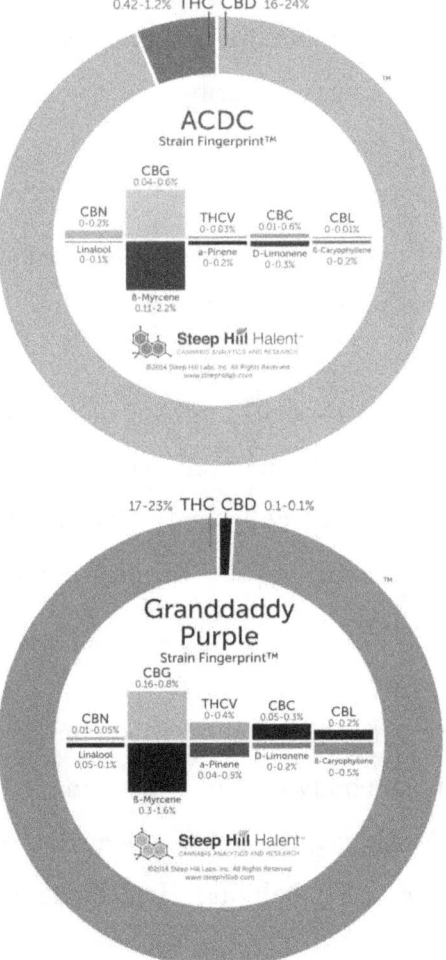

Stuart Cameron
Patterson, NY

Stuart Cameron, 62, lives in a leafy hamlet in upper Westchester County, NY. Recently remarried to Laurie, he has been wrestling with Parkinson's since 1996. It was six years of waking up, wondering, "What's next?": It's been more than another decade of waking up every morning, wondering how to shake it off and have a good day.

It's easy to forget, or not to know at all, that Parkinson's strikes us in our so-called prime.

Stuart was a high school English teacher in New Hampshire. Early on, he tried to disguise the symptoms from his friends and colleagues. But by 2004, the symptoms became too prevalent, and Stu retired on disability.

He was then regularly falling down, the result of the dyskinesia, his body no longer listening to his commands. The depression was weighing on him. The tremors were overwhelming. He considered the options for an "exit" plan. Discussing the plan with his teenage daughter, she said, "I understand…completely."

Desperate, he agreed to have a Deep Brain Stimulator (DBS) implanted. This was a grueling, eight-hour surgery that required him to be awake the entire time.

The DBS helped regain some stability and control of his limbs. But six years later, on a normal day, he felt a sharp charge of electricity in his brain and he passed out. Upon waking he realized he'd lost his peripheral vision. Like a broken toy, a wire corroded inside his brain, causing a short circuit.

The DBS had to be removed. An infection ensued, which required several brain operations. (It takes me three seconds to type, "several brain operations." The hospitalizations took considerably longer,) He chose not to have a new one installed. Stu had been a recreational user of pot. Living in New York, he wasn't eligible for medical marijuana. But now his ex-wife suggested he try, just to relieve the pain.

"It took me away from the pain. It took my mind away

from the pain."

These days he smokes four or five times a week, getting marijuana from the underground. It relieves his restless leg syndrome and general malaise, and enables him to stretch, and, yes, disregard the pain.

His drug portfolio includes a handful of doctor-prescribed medicine. Marijuana is simply part of the regimen.

"Why? I know my body well."

This enables him to engage in carpentry, a lifelong interest. And his wife, Laurie, says, "Today he's painting the exterior of the house. He might even come in from the rain."

Patients come for the cannabis and stay for the medicine.

Laurie Cameron
Patterson, NY

If Laurie Cameron were a pill that came in a bottle it would be green and brown because Laurie is earthy, but without the dirt. She's serious and fun, usually at the exact same moment.

Laurie married Stuart Cameron three years ago, second marriages for both. Stu already had Parkinson's for more than a decade.

"It's lonely being a spouse. But I refuse to let Parkinson's take over our lives. It's not that we don't giggle and have fun. We do. But without marijuana he can shut down."

Shutting down can mean disengaging from the things that make Stu, Stu: reading, painting, and fixing stuff.

"Marijuana lifts the Parkinson's 'mask' he's been assigned to wear. Parkinson's makes him withdraw into himself; he even looks different," she told me.

"It screws with your mind and your body."

But the marijuana brings Stu back to "normal." We agree that's not high, not low, just smack in the middle. Yet Stu doesn't get high during the day, perhaps because it's cultural, like waiting until 5pm to have the first cocktail. If so, Laurie agrees it's crazy:

"Marijuana is medicine. It doesn't even look like a martini. And unlike so much Western medicine that takes weeks for you to know if it's working before you try some other medicine… Marijuana works right away."

"I like right away."

She concludes, if only for now: "Plus it makes the journey less lonely, I get to reclaim him. And it makes him 'even.' Not giddy, not silly. But come to think of it, I'd take silly."

Chapter

11

M or C: Marijuana or Cannabis?

In the course of researching this book the authors discovered a language fence. The fence, while not impenetrable, is in our minds, a waste of resources and a little like all fences: it prompts people to ask, "Why did they bother putting it up?"

"Marijuana"

Marijuana can be a radioactive word. It was born in fear and probably racism. When the U.S. government wanted its citizens to steer clear of marijuana early in the 20th century, it blamed Mexicans for bringing it across southern borders and infecting our population.

The use of the word "marijuana" became entirely associated with recreation and criminal or outlaw behavior: dangerous, anti-social, the gateway to even more dangerous and addictive drugs.

So in an effort to restore marijuana to its origins as an herbal medicine, many practitioners, dispensaries, and well-meaning organizations are trying to eradicate use of the M word in favor of the C word.

"Cannabis"

Yes, cannabis is the Latin word for the actual plant, so the word is certainly authentic. It doesn't have all the pejorative baggage that "marijuana" has.

But real people, the patients and their families, legislators and the media, persist in saying marijuana. That's what they know, that's what they're comfortable saying.

It's tough enough to get people to change their attitudes and behavior when everything is crystal clear. The language fight actually sows confusion among some people when they learn that cannabis is marijuana.

It's really a waste of time, energy, and resources. And it's also elitist. Let's stick to helping people feel and get better as opposed to trying to rebrand a product or medicine.

Marijuana = Cannabis

People are going to say what they want to say. This isn't about comparing apples to oranges. It's all apples. Let's stop trying to correct them. Let's focus on making them feel better.

Marijuana

=

Cannabis

Jeffrey Hergenrather, M.D.
Sebastopol, CA

Many of Jeff Hergenrather's patients think of him as the hippie doctor and for good reason. Jeff graduated from U.C.-Berkeley and Brown Medical School. Yes, he smoked marijuana in college, recreationally. But it wasn't until he was a doctor, practicing on "The Farm," a commune in south-central Tennessee, that he discovered the benefits of medical marijuana.

It was there that he learned, along with other doctors, that cannabis was a safe form of treatment for a variety of ailments. He, too, had learned of the endocannabinoid system as one of the body's methods to maintain homeostasis, but didn't see its practical applications until he was on the Farm.

And like many doctors and patients, using marijuana became personal for him. His son, Sammy, suffered a diving accident, and became a quadriplegic, but remained cognitively intact. Moving the family to California for better care, Jeff settled into Sebastopol, a progressive community of farmers. Understanding that medical marijuana could aid his son's uncontrolled muscle spasms, he asked Sam's doctor to prescribe it. When the doctor refused, fearing the radioactive PR, Jeff prescribed it himself.

The success was immediate, such that many of Sammy's friends at rehab came to Jeff for prescriptions, too. That's how he became a medical marijuana doctor, with over 2,200 patients, most who come back, for treatment beyond the medical marijuana.

"Marijuana helps the patient eat, sleep, detox, and protect. The endocannabinoid system facilitates the destruction of harmful cells." In addition to the indica and sativa strains, he is optimistic about the current research underway in Japan, China, and Israel regarding the role of terpenes, organic compounds that produce a distinctive smell and taste in things like marijuana, wine and essential oils.

"And when the drug war against medical marijuana ends – and it will – we will learn all its healing properties as we now know just some." Jeff believes medical marijuana benefits the adaptogens in the body that maintain our homeostasis. This means the body knows what it needs and is able to extract from the medical marijuana just that.

Homeostasis is the body's ability to maintain internal stability in the wake of external changes like temperature.

For instance, if our body needs to rest and we ingest a sativa strain that would normally make us more alert and creative, a needed effect – sleep – would more likely result because that's what the body needs.

Smart body. Smart marijuana.

Smart body.

Smart marijuana.

Chapter

12

Is it just US?

A great number of Americans simply are uninterested in what transpires outside America. This may be especially true about politics – which can be wearying and depressing – as well as about culture, art, and even medicine.

This attitude is a product of our sense of self-importance as Americans, and our belief the world revolves around us. And it's also a function of the "just leave me alone" attitude.

But if you're interested in medical marijuana and have gotten this far in the book, it's safe to assume you're not that type of person. Rather, you want to know both other American citizens' experiences and other world citizens' experiences, too.

Canada

Medical marijuana is legal in Canada. But the benefits only extend to a few thousand patients due to a labyrinth of laws and regulations. Many patients still face criminal prosecution. Despite Canada's – or because of – Canada's Marijuana Medical Access

Regulations (MMAR), patients need sworn statements by physicians pretty much declaring "all else has failed"; licenses to grow their own marijuana or designees who are authorized in their behalf; The MMAR includes other onerous rules to prevent widespread medical use. So it's hardly surprising that millions go their own quasi-legal way and choose compassion clubs that skirt the laws.

Netherlands

The Dutch legalized the sale of marijuana forty years ago. One can buy it, freely, in stores called coffee shops. (Yes, they also sell coffee. Imagine Starbucks' stock price if they did, too.) Pharmacies also dispense marijuana by prescription. The Dutch probably have the most liberal marijuana laws in the Western world. So you would expect that a greater number of its citizens would be regular marijuana users than, say, Americans. Surprise: More than twice the percentage of Americans report using marijuana in the past month.

Marijuana Usage

2013	Used Past Month (Age 15+)	
	U.S.	Netherlands
Cannabis	**9.4%**	**4.2%**

Source: 2013 National Survey on Drug Use and Health (NSDUH)
2014 European Monitoring Centre for Drugs and Drug Addiction

Obviously, this is but one statistic plucked from two enormous reports. But the meaning is apparent: prohibition doesn't reduce usage; rather, it likely encourages it.

Israel

Medical marijuana has been legal in Israel since the 1960s, though recreational use is still prohibited. Israel is one of the leading countries conducting research into the medical benefits of marijuana. Israeli scientists Raphael Mechoulam and Yechiel Gaoni were the first to isolate THC in marijuana in 1964. And in what can surely be described as a progressive move, the Israeli Army prescribes medical marijuana for PTSD.

China

Despite the fact that hemp is a very important crop in China, marijuana is very illegal. The same is true of Japan, where, the US created the law there following World War II.

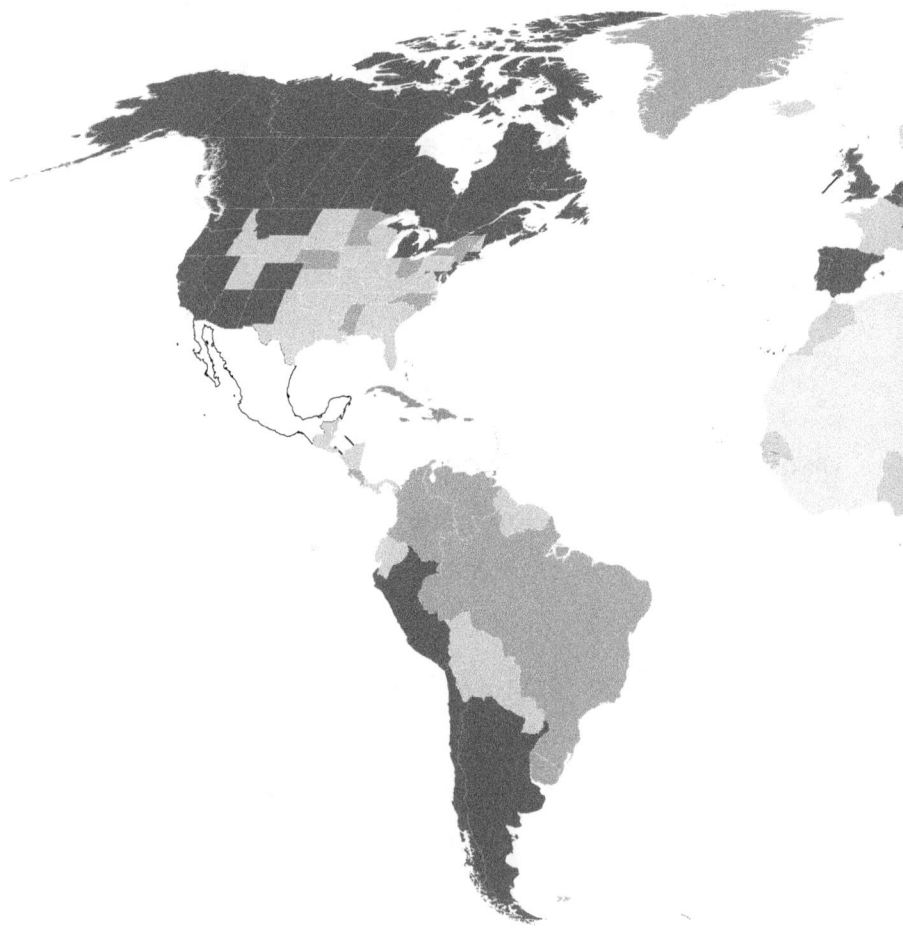

Marijuana Legalization Status

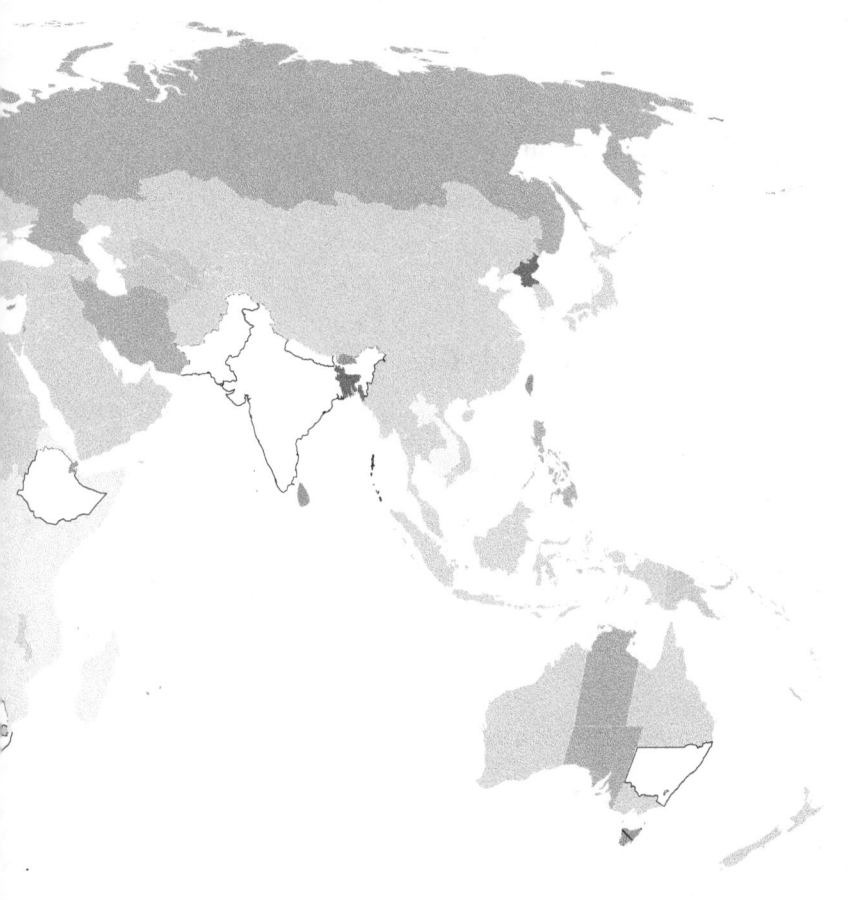

- Legal / Essentially Legal
- Decriminalized
- Illegal, but often unenforced
- Illegal
- No information

Dustin Sulak, D.O.
Manchester, ME

Dustin Sulak, 35, grew up suspecting he wasn't told the whole truth about health and healing. He recalls suffering from a number of chronic illnesses as a teenager. He was treated by allopathic medicine – what we would call "normal" medicine with "doctors and pills" – which he said actually made him worse. This experience opened him to the possibilities of homeopathic treatment, methods that work with the body as opposed to attacking it.

After college he enrolled at the Arizona College of Osteopathy. During a pharmacology lecture he learned about the endocannabinoid system and became fascinated by the relationship of botany with medicine. Dustin was particularly influenced by John McPartland, an endocannabinoid researcher.

Sulak is one of the founders of Maine Integrative Health, which has offices in Portland, Augusta, and Massachusetts. They have 18,000 patients, 99% of who use cannabis, Sulak considers marijuana as a gateway drug, but not the gateway you're accustomed to hearing.

Patients come for the cannabis and stay for the medicine.

That medicine includes therapy, osteopathy, hypnotherapy, yoga, nutrition, and reiki. But Sulak doesn't rest on his current knowledge.

He regularly attends conferences and learns about new treatments and disciplines. He spent time training with a Lakota Medicine Chief and a Lubavitcher Rabbi.

Chapter

13

What's next: Optimism.

When we began this book the readers and the authors probably had something interesting in common: we didn't know a heck of a lot about medical marijuana.

We employed an iterative process, in which we researched, wrote, researched more, and wrote some more. Then we went back over the manuscript to be sure we didn't say dumb stuff earlier on.

The research, of course, included already published sources, which are named at the end of the book. But the "real" research, the primary research where we actually learned what the medical marijuana landscape looks like in late 2014 was gained by interviewing the people who are most directly involved with patient care:

The doctors and the patients.

It seems like an appropriate time to ask the question, "What exactly have we learned?"

Medical marijuana makes sick people normal.

Patients overwhelmingly report that they use medical marijuana to function as normal people.

The appreciation of normal seems to only arrive in its absence.

Medical marijuana isn't about getting high.

It's about getting "medium," smack in the middle of high and low.

Medical marijuana relieves, eliminates, provides, alleviates...

- By relieving chronic pain without opioids

- By eliminating chronic seizures

- Provides a decent night's sleep

- By reducing the rigidity of Parkinson's

- By alleviating the depression associated with

  chronic illness

- By enabling us to work, play, and even enjoy life

Medical marijuana can be the ticket for patients to return to being people.

How did Laurie Cameron phrase it?

"Marijuana lifts the Parkinson's mask my husband Stu has been forced to wear."

Medical marijuana is personal.

So many of the doctors, patients, and activists who appear in the book were introduced to medical marijuana through illnesses they or members of their family have endured.

Medical marijuana is still contro- versial.

Practitioners cannot prescribe marijuana in the open even in states where it is entirely legal.

They are still hounded by state licensing boards, other doctors and Not in My Backyard neighbors, police, and politicians.

Employees cannot tell colleagues, managers, or HR for fear of increased scrutiny or even dismissal.

Bosses can't tell employees for fear of lost respect and control. (And you thought it would be impossible to feel bad for bosses.)

Medical marijuana can be the gateway to good medicine.

A discovery of medical marijuana often leads to other "alternative" therapies to help patients who have been disappointed, or maybe abandoned, by Western medicine.

This includes but isn't limited to acupuncture, yoga, reiki, and other herbal medicine.

Medical marijuana is still confused with recreational marijuana.

It isn't unusual for non-patients to snicker at the concept of "medical" marijuana, given the far greater awareness of marijuana as a recreational drug.

It's easy to dismiss medical marijuana as just an excuse to get high if that's all someone has learned.

You now have the tools and even privilege of straightening people out, one at a time.

Medical marijuana is still a Schedule I Drug.

There are surely greater injustices than being a Schedule I drug.

But for marijuana to be in the same category as heroin, this injustice is right up there.

Medical marijuana usage is still against federal law.

Individual states can enact their own "Compassionate Care" laws making medical marijuana legal. Since 1996, twenty-six states and the District of Columbia have done so. The federal government rarely prosecutes individual patients in these states.

That's a good thing. But it's still illegal. And they retain the right and power to do so.

Or they did until December 13, 2014 when the U.S. Senate passed a budget that eliminated all funding of federal prosecution of marijuana cases in states where medical marijuana is legal.

By taking away the funding the US Department of Justice will no longer raid, prosecute or incarcerate.

Medical marijuana still needs more research.

We don't fear research: We applaud it. As the government reduces its stranglehold on legal supply (remember the Mississippi lab and vault that has monopolistic control?), more doctors and scientists will be able to determine the full extent of the benefits and, yes, the question marks of medical marijuana.

For instance: the December 2014 issue of Neurology Reviews reported on the research presented at the 43rd Annual Meeting of the Child Neurology Society. There, Francis M. Filloux, MD, Chief of the Division of Pediatric Neurology at the University of Utah School of Medicine warned of the possibility of "the opportunity [marijuana has] to mess up motor function and coordination, and have a major impact on mood and behavioral regulation."

(The patients we interviewed would surely agree with the impact on mood. Just not in the direction Dr. Filloux is thinking about.)

Yet as Dr. Filloux summarized, "Certain marijuana products are probably effective in treating MS, clearly effective in treating pain and nausea, and generating excitement about a possible benefit in certain types of childhood epilepsy."

And he concluded, "There is no doubt that in the next year or two, we'll have a lot more information." Until then, you can decide if medical marijuana is appropriate for you and your loved ones.

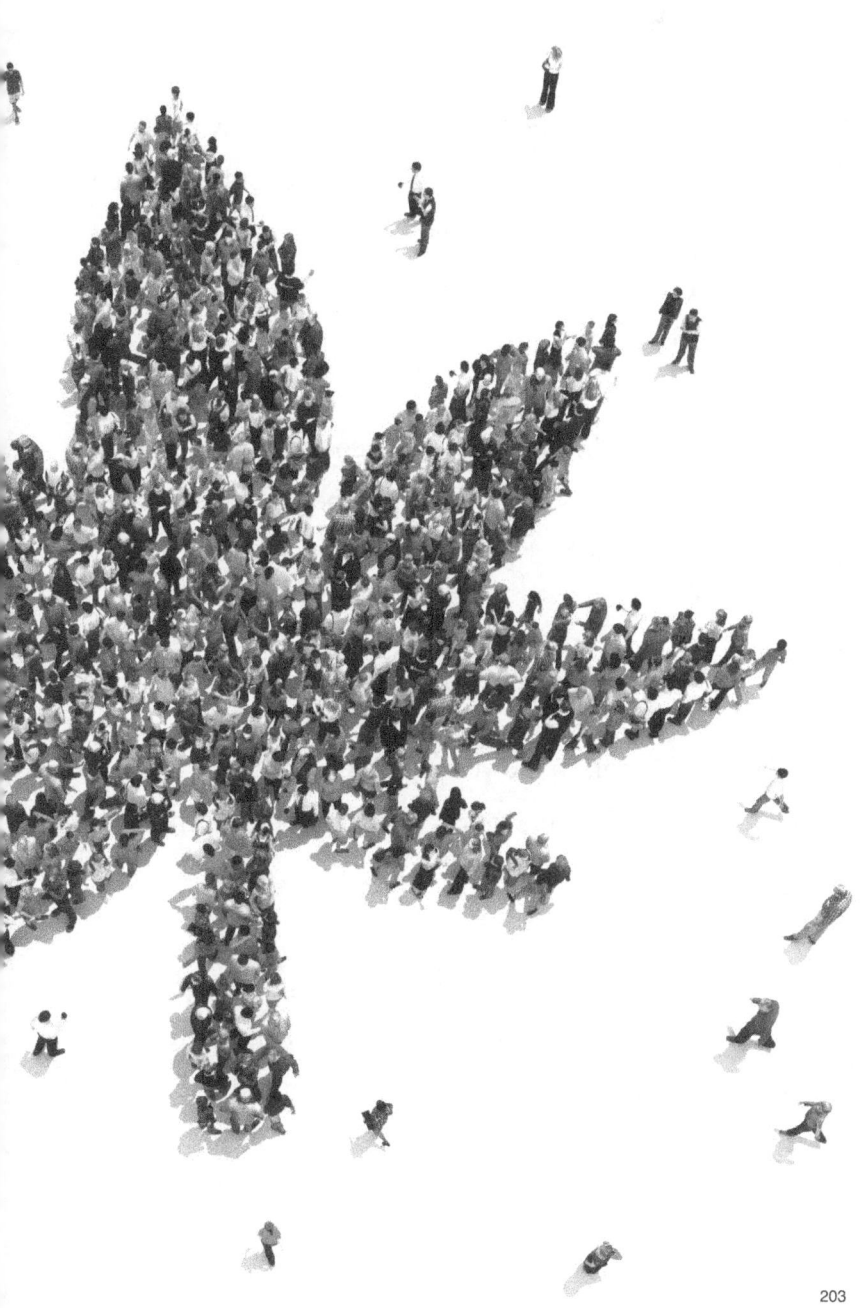

Tom Macy
Chatham, MA

Tom Macy (not his real name) is a business owner in Cape Cod, Massachusetts. Tom, 44, thought he grew up in a normal household. Except his mother suffered from a bipolar disorder, so little was really normal about his childhood.

It all came to a head a few years ago when he contracted arthritis in his legs. This began a litany of painkillers and anti-depressants and dependency.

Talking to Tom I'm reminded about a statistic I had recently seen released by the Centers for Disease Control. In the year 2012 there were 16,000 deaths in the U.S. due to narcotic (opioid) painkiller overdoses. That's 44 people a day, every day.

Tom, however, had the good fortune to get into therapy. There he learned the arthritis was just the gift-wrapping for his PTSD of coping with a sick mom his entire childhood.

With the unrelenting support of his wife, Kate, he made his way to the Maine Integrative Health office in Burlington, MA. Under the care of Dr. Joseph Rottman (who passed away in October, 2014), Tom was able to kick the narcotics.

"I'm down to one-half a Klonopin a day." He previously needed three whole pills.

Instead, he vapes an Indica blend a few times a day and practices yoga. He says his new regimen saved not only his business but his life. "I was in the throes of addiction. I'm proud to say I'm highly functional. I know some people say medical marijuana is a gateway drug. Well, I say it's an exit from pain."

Suggested reading and resources.

The Pot Book, edited by Julie Holland, M.D., Park Street Press

Marijuana, Reconsidered, Lester Grinspoon, M.D., Cahners Business Press

Marijuana Medical Handbook. Practical Guide to Therapeutic Use of Marijuana, Gregory T. Carter, Quick American Archives

Americans for Safe Access
www.safeaccessnow.org

Cannabis Patients Alliance
www.cannabispatients.org

Law Enforcement Against Prohibition (LEAP)
www.leap.cc

National Organization for the Reform of Marijuana Laws (NORML)
www.norml.org

Realm of Caring

theroc.us

Patients out of Time

www.medicalcannabis.com

Acknowledgements.

All the patients who trusted me with their stories are attributed in Pot Luck except for the few who regretfully couldn't. All the doctors named here, are fighting the good fight, against censure and discrimination and threat of suspension, especially Lester Grinspoon, M.D., who not so many years ago began to despair that he would never see the end of the destructive prohibition in his lifetime, but is now dazzled by the rapidity with which it's becoming a reality.

All those who connected me to more people: Julie Holland, M.D., Jeff Hergenrather, M.D., Dustin Sulak, D.O., Larry Lonky, O.D., Amy Richer, Hunter Holliman, Americans for Safe Access, and Allison Ray Benavides, Realm of Caring, California.

The manuscript readers who insured the science is science; and prevented me from writing inelegantly, but also want to keep their day jobs.

Juergen Dahlen, chief honcho of DahlenDesign,
my friend and creative force behind RL Books,
who designs a book that appears to be worth reading.

Finally, Isabel, who keeps me on the straight and
narrow.